LIVING WITHOUT PAIN

ARTHRITIS
FIBROMYALGIA
LUPUS
CHRONIC FATIGUE SYNDROME

THEIR CAUSE

AND HOW TO OVERCOME THEM

NATURALLY!

"Being *FIT FOR LIFE* means being *PAIN-FREE FOR LIFE*"

Harvey Diamond

Co-author of the *New York Times* Bestseller *FIT FOR LIFE*
Over 12 Million Copies Sold

ISBN: 0-9769961-0-3

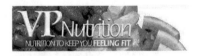

VP Nutrition Inc.
P.O. Box 188
Osprey , Florida 34229
www.vpnutrition.com
877-335-1509

This book was printed in the U.S.A.
The Feeling Fit Group®/877-335-1509   info@vpnutrition.com

05 06 07 08 09 10   5 4 3 2

"We certainly cannot succeed as a culture by continuing to deny and ignore pain, as if we could silence it beneath a mountain of pills."

—*David Morris*

TABLE OF CONTENTS

PART ONE—THE DILEMMA

PART TWO—THE SOLUTION

PART ONE

THE DILEMMA

INTRODUCTION

To live life free of pain; now there's a tantalizing prospect if ever there was one. But is it possible? Is it possible to live one's life without a seemingly never ending procession of annoying and troublesome aches and pains, some minor, some major, that appear to plague us relentlessly from the cradle to the grave? Well yes, of course it's **possible**, but from all available indications it certainly doesn't seem probable. After all, when you examine the statistics associated with pain it is glaringly obvious that pain in America is increasingly becoming more common, not less so.

In 1985 a Louis Harris Poll revealed that pain was the number one health complaint in the United States.[1] What's happened since then? The latest Gallup Poll most assuredly reinforces the assertion that pain, the "hidden epidemic," is America's number one public health problem[2] The numbers are so striking it's difficult to grasp the full measure of the problem. Nine out of ten adults (89%) suffer from pain on some kind of regular basis (at least once a month).[3] More startling is the fact that a whopping **42%** endure pain **every single day**[4]

Percentages are one thing; it's when you look at the actual number of people who are affected by pain that you begin to fully appreciate the true scope of the problem. Forty-two percent of the adult population translates into over 90 million people who are in pain every day without letup. For one third of these sufferers, their chronic pain is so severe and debilitating, they feel they can't function as normal people and sometimes it is so bad they want to die![5] Is it any wonder the survey revealed that 80% of Americans believe that pain is simply a part of getting older[6] with 60% stating that pain was something you simply had to learn to live with?[7] A surprising 28% indicated that they felt there was no solution for them and nothing could be done for their pain.[8]

The National Institute of Health estimates that pain costs us over $100 billion a year in medical expenses, lost wages and other costs.[9] Stating that chronic pain was the most urgent and ignored health issue in the United States, exasperated, Congressman Mike Rogers (R-MI), in April 2003, introduced **H.R. 1863**, *the National Pain Care Policy Act of 2003* in the House of Representatives. His bill was designed to not only improve public awareness and understanding of the plight of those who deal with unrelenting pain everyday but also to allocate more resources for pain research.

What about you; what's your belief system about pain? Are you one of the 170 million or so people who have bought into the inevitability of pain? Are you convinced that because it's so prevalent it's just a matter of time before something starts to hurt? True, pain **is** widespread, but what about the more than 50 million adults who do **not** experience pain regularly? How do they manage to beat the odds? Obviously it is possible to do so because so many people **are** living their lives free of pain. How is that explained? Is it their lifestyle? Does it have to do with their diet, whether or not they exercise, whether they smoke or drink alcohol? Is it that they were blessed with good genes? Is it their positive or negative attitude toward life? Is it simply good fortune? Or is it a combination of all of these factors?

Having studied this subject intensely for 35 years I am convinced beyond any possible doubt that being hounded by pain with increasing frequency and severity as time goes by is **not** part of life's grand scheme. Notwithstanding the striking number of people who do have to contend with pain on a regular basis, living pain free is the normal and natural condition of the human body and is what the living body itself strives for with unwavering resolve. Although pain does, under certain circumstances, serve a vital purpose, which I will clearly explain later, unrelenting pain is completely abnormal and unnatural.

If you are at all familiar with any of my previous books then you know that the primary reason why I decided to dedicate myself to the study of health was because I was in excruciating, unrelenting pain that dogged me every day of my life for over 20 years. After learning how to naturally overcome that pain and prevent its return, the results of an unintentional poisoning of my body with a horribly toxic chemical very nearly killed me and brought another several-year bout of daily pain into my life. Once again, without the use of a single drug, I was victorious over the pain. Today I am in my sixties and I live pain free. No stomachaches, no headaches, no back pain, no muscle pain, no joint pain—no pain! And don't think that I am not thrilled about **that**.

My personal experiences certainly disprove the majority belief that as one ages, pain becomes an ever increasing likelihood. It is just the opposite with me. Not because I'm special or lucky or different from anyone reading this right now but because I was fortunate enough to come into contact with the information that would help me conquer pain and I had the good sense to utilize it. By reading this book you are also going to have that exact same opportunity. I hope with all my heart that you will give it a fair trial and find out for yourself, as I did, that overcoming pain and preventing its return is something that you are in charge of rather than circumstances that are outside of your control.

It would be an understatement of the highest order to point out that the nature of pain has been sorrowfully misunderstood. The unrecognized truth of the matter is that pain has a purpose, a cause, and a remedy. This fact has somehow eluded the medical community which has regrettably resulted in a host of assertions that cannot be proven and illogical speculation that borders on the absurd. The consequence of this misinterpretation of pain has led to the tragic reliance on drugs as the lone solution of choice; highly toxic drugs that do absolutely nothing to remove the underlying cause of the pain and are used only in an attempt to render the symptoms more tolerable. This ill-fated strategy certainly helps explain why pain continues to be the number one health complaint in the United States with no letup in sight.

Let me state clearly here at the onset that I do not claim to have the answer to every painful condition that can befall the human body. The plain and honest truth is that there are a number of variables, some known some unknown, which can be a factor in why a person is in pain. For me to assert that regardless of those variables, all someone in pain has to do is follow the recommendations found herein and the pain will go away would be naïve and frankly, dishonest. I do not wish to mislead or to sugar coat my message giving the impression that this is the be-all and end-all when it comes to overcoming pain.

What I will tell you with complete sincerity and confidence is this: there are four terribly painful and debilitating conditions that affect millions upon millions of people every single day with which I am very familiar and have had a considerable amount of success in guiding people to overcome. The four conditions I am referring to are Fibromyalgia, Lupus, Arthritis and Chronic Fatigue Syndrome. Again, I don't wish to imply that anyone suffering from these particular maladies is guaranteed success in overcoming them regardless of individual circumstances that would prevent their successful removal. But rest assured, based on my previous experience with people, millions may well be helped and others could at the very least see a significant lessening of their symptoms.

There is a very definite reason why this book focuses primarily on Fibromyalgia, Lupus, Arthritis, and Chronic Fatigue Syndrome and the reason might surprise you. In fact you are likely to read certain things here that are so diametrically opposed to what you have heard in the past that your first inclination might be to toss the book aside with a comment about my grasp on reality. There will undoubtedly be those "experts" who take issue with my premise but success leaves clues, and different though my take may be, people have had success following the recommendations you are about to read.

You should bear in mind that over the course of far too many years, in the face of so many millions of people suffering every day with the number continuing to rise, and billions and billions of dollars being spent on research and treatment, not the slightest, most infinitesimal glimmer of headway has been made in alleviating these maladies. That is unless you classify a boatload of new, expensive drugs designed only to fight the symptoms as headway. All these problems have done is get worse and destroy people's lives. Of **course** something new and revolutionary, not the same old party line, is what is needed if we are to have some progress; and that is exactly what you will find within these pages.

Fibromyalgia, Lupus, and Arthritis are essentially the same malady as far as the living body is concerned and Chronic Fatigue Syndrome is, more often than not, one of the results of those conditions. To say it even more accurately, Fibromyalgia, Lupus, and Arthritis are the same malady being differentiated only by where in the body they occur. Although one can have Chronic Fatigue Syndrome and not have Fibromyalgia, Lupus, or Arthritis, it is extremely common for it to occur along with them.

So, if as I suggest, Fibromyalgia, Lupus, Arthritis, and Chronic Fatigue Syndrome are connected, what is it then that differentiates one from the other? Not much, as it turns out. In fact, they have more similarities than differences.

1. All four are referred to as auto-immune diseases.

2. All four are extremely debilitating.

3. All four are associated with inflammation in the body. (This is a huge bone of contention in that Fibromyalgia is not considered to be so, but as you shall see, it certainly is.)

4. All four are considered by the medical profession to be caused by mysterious and unknown factors.

5. All four are treated with drugs to quell the symptoms.

6. All four have the exact same cause.

7. All four have the exact same remedy.

Throughout the course of this book the seven points made above will be discussed in much greater detail, especially numbers six and seven. The book is divided into two parts. Part one is the dilemma, and the much larger part two is the solution, the part I'm sure you are most interested in. Am I right?

For now I want to tell you that your days of suffering are about to be relieved. Right about now I can understand if you are saying something to the effect of, "From your lips to God's ears; please let it be so." I don't make the statement that your suffering is soon to be lessened lightly. For the many millions of people who have to deal with the symptoms of Fibromyalgia,

Lupus, Arthritis, and Chronic Fatigue Syndrome, I am familiar, as I am sure you are, with the long list of frustrations that you have to contend with every day.

First and foremost on the list of frustrations associated with these conditions is, unquestionably, pain. Except perhaps for some misguided masochists, no one likes pain. Even intermittent, on-again, off-again pain is debilitating and disruptive to one's lifestyle. But the pain associated with Fibromyalgia, Lupus, Arthritis, and Chronic Fatigue Syndrome is frequently severe and unrelenting, which tends to drain the joy right out of life, making it a chore to enjoy even the simplest of activities that most people take completely for granted.

Added to the incessant pain is the further frustration of being told by the medical community that it is entirely baffled about the cause or origin of Fibromyalgia, Lupus, Arthritis, and Chronic Fatigue Syndrome, and the only course of action it can recommend is an experimental drugging campaign in the hope that it can somehow reduce the symptoms. Essentially, being told that there is no hope in sight and the best that can be expected is to find drugs that will reduce the symptoms without harming you further is no way to live. I am telling you that you don't have to live that way, and I wrote this book to prove it to you.

Having gone through what I know you have if you are reading this book looking for answers, I completely understand if you are having feelings of skepticism that I, a person working basically on his own, outside the vast medical community, have come up with the answers that have thus far eluded the medical doctors. Frankly, I don't blame you. Knowing me, if I were in your position I would be skeptical too. All I ask is that you give what I have to say a fair hearing and a fair trial. You won't be sorry.

Since this is the introduction, perhaps I can very briefly introduce myself and give you insight into how I can declare with such certainty that the information contained in this book can help you. Let me assure you that it did not come about "overnight". Not by a longshot.

I have been around the sun now 60 times, and for 35 of those 60 years I have been studying and teaching the principles of good health. I am profoundly touched and exceedingly gratified that my work, through my books, has helped improve the health and lives of literally millions of people around the world. The **FIT FOR LIFE** books have sold over 12 million copies in 33 languages and are read in over 80 countries.

I did not start out with the idea of healing the world's ills. On the contrary, I started studying health for strictly selfish reasons. I was in desperate need of something to help me overcome a host of health problems, most prominently an excruciatingly painful condition that was medicated for over two decades, all to no avail. Plus, I watched helplessly as my father died of cancer of the stomach (and its treatment) after suffering for years with many of the same complaints I had.

In 1970, at age 25, I made the commitment to study health so I could recapture my own health and live out my life without pain, ill health, and disease. I quickly decided against entering the medical profession because, as it turns out, the entire $1.6 trillion-a-year[10] medical profession is set up for the express purpose of treating people **after** they're sick. You don't go to the doctor when you're well, do you? The main subject of study for a medical student is pathology—the study of disease. Do you happen to know the word in the English language for the study of health? **There isn't one!**

Fortunately for me and millions of other people, I came across an almost entirely unknown field of study called **Natural Hygiene.** Even though it has a nearly 200-year written history, most people had never heard of it—including me. Unlike the medical profession, it is based on studying the prerequisites of health, not only to recapture health, but also to do what is necessary to maintain it. In other words, it's what you do when you're well to see to it that you stay that way.

The basis of Natural Hygiene is that the human body is self-repairing, self-healing, and self-maintaining. It is incomprehensibly intelligent and is supremely capable of healing itself of any malady whatsoever, no matter how seemingly complex, if—and this is a great, big, humungous if—**IF** it is given the opportunity to do so.

What attracted me to Natural Hygiene was that it was so straightforward, obvious, and logical. Unlike the medical profession, which shrugs its shoulders and declares that it has no answers, Natural Hygiene answers all questions pertaining to health and ill health in an easy-to-understand, common sense fashion that resonates with truth that is easy to verify in one's life simply by putting the principles into practice; which is exactly what I did. Following years of medical jargon and doublespeak that shed no light whatsoever on my painful condition and left me feeling in the dark about what was going on, I felt so liberated to finally have a reasonable, understandable explanation and some common sense principles to apply that would bring me relief.

After I applied these principles, what seemed like magic happened in my life. Not only did the painful disorder that I had to endure **every day** for over 20 years simply disappear, never to return again, but my perennial lack of energy that left me feeling like a sloth slogging through quicksand was replaced by an astounding energy level that some of my friends found to be annoying. I discovered in myself a newfound exuberance for life that I had begun to think I would never experience.

That's when I decided that I wanted to make the study and teaching of the principles of Natural Hygiene my life's work. At that time (early 1970s) only one school in the United States offered a complete course in Natural Hygiene. Although it was a non-accredited school (what a surprise, the medical profession didn't acknowledge it), the curriculum was extensive and highly comprehensive. I devoured it. Over the next two years I completed the entire course and was awarded a Ph.D. in Nutritional Science. I continued studying on my own and read all that I could on Natural Hygiene, which was a considerable body of work.

Then it was time to share the good news with the world. As an added, and much welcomed, benefit of using the principles referred to above to vanquish the pain from my life and skyrocket my energy levels, I also lost 50 pounds of unwanted weight I had been wrestling with for several years. I decided to write a book based on the principles of Natural Hygiene to help people lose weight.

The first **FIT FOR LIFE** book was published in 1985[11], and it was an immediate sensation. At a record-breaking pace it ascended to the top of the bestseller lists. And it stayed there. It held the coveted #1 position on the *New York Times* Best-seller List for an unprecedented 40 straight weeks—a record it still holds. Due to its no nonsense, straightforward, time-less, and effective principles, 20 years later it still sells 100,000 copies a year worldwide.

The result of that book's phenomenal success first ignited in me an interest and understanding of Fibromyalgia, Lupus, Arthritis, and Chronic Fatigue Syndrome. By the time the early to mid-1990s had rolled around I had received over 500,000 letters from people sharing the success they had enjoyed as a result of reading **FIT FOR LIFE**—everything from over-coming the mildest of conditions all the way to, and including, cancer. Some of the stories were so inspir-ing they brought tears to the eye. Nothing could have been a greater validation of the effectiveness of the principles of Natural Hygiene than these letters.

With ever increasing regularity, I started to hear of success stories regarding Fibromyalgia, Lupus, Arthritis, and Chronic Fatigue Syndrome. Actually, I was already well acquainted with Chronic Fatigue Syndrome because the first and most quickly recog-nizable result of utilizing the principles I'm referring to is an obvious and dramatic increase in one's level of energy. And since more people commented on one aspect or another of their newfound energy than on any other subject, I was all too familiar with conditions that were the result of a habitual lack of energy. To this day it is the one thing people comment on more frequently than any other.

Although I also had a good understanding of Arthritis, in all honesty, I was only slightly familiar with Fibromyalgia or Lupus. But as more and more people started sharing with me that they had finally found something that actually worked in helping them feel better, I made it my business to learn more. Frankly, I was stunned to learn how many millions of people worldwide suffer from Fibromyalgia and Lupus. What did not surprise me in the least was the fact that one of the most common co-existing conditions associated with Fibromyalgia and Lupus is Chronic Fatigue Syndrome. In fact, some estimates say that a diagnosis of Fibromyalgia and Chronic Fatigue Syndrome is interchangeable.[12] What you will find out as you read the book, is that Fibromyalgia, Lupus, and Arthritis contribute to a lack of energy, and the lack of energy prevents the symptoms of Fibromyalgia, Lupus, and Arthritis from abating.

This is the eighth book I have written. The principles of Natural Hygiene are utilized in all as the backdrop for whatever objective I attempt to convey in each book. This book takes the very best of all I have ever learned as it relates specifically to understanding and overcoming Fibromyalgia, Lupus, Arthritis, and Chronic Fatigue Syndrome.

What the contents of this book offer you is a reasonable and doable strategy for success. Not with a hit or miss approach that depends on dangerous drugs or some magical potion; not with actions that fly in the face of reason; but with an understandable and sensible game plan that honors the extraordinary living body and works in harmony with and in concert with the intelligence that governs every activity of the body.

An intelligence is at work in the Universe—that is self-evident. And this intelligence that is completely beyond our ability to fully comprehend **knows what it's doing!** This intelligence knew how to hurl all the stars and planets into space in such an orderly fashion. One look around at the splendor and grandeur that is everywhere to be seen in the natural world, and it is impossible not to marvel at the indescribable intelligence that governs it all. We can only stand in humble awe of its magnificence. This unparalleled intelligence is at work in your body right now!

People have lots of different names that they use to describe this intelligence I'm talking about. Some call it God, Mother Nature, The Grand Creator, The Life Force. All work for me, and I use them all. I'm partial to the word *God*, because for me it encompasses everything—but that's me. Now I would never be so foolhardy as to attempt to tell you what God is or what you should think God is; it's way too personal a subject. I wouldn't think of trying to push my beliefs about God on you or try to change your personal views on the subject. But I **will** say that whenever I mention God, you will know I am referring to that Supreme Intelligence I have been discussing. Whatever special, unique, and personal feelings you have in your heart about God, that's what I'm talking about.

Having said that, I want to tell you that God would never drop us onto this planet, make us susceptible to every possible malady imaginable, and not also provide us with what we need to overcome them. No way. God is far more kind and loving than that. Everything you need to live a highly energetic, pain-free life is available to you. It's just a matter of uncovering it and using it. I want to instill in you a brand-new reverence, admiration, and respect for your body and the forces that preside over its well-being. We live in a cause-and-effect universe. Things don't just happen to you, they happen as a result of actions you took earlier. It may not appear to be so at first glance, but absolutely **everything** regarding your well-being is unfolding in an orderly and organized fashion. It may appear to be haphazard circumstances that bring on pain and ill health, but it's not. Pain and a consistent lack of energy are the direct result of either doing something to your body that you shouldn't have done or not doing something for your body that you should have done.

Health is the normal, natural state of your body. Ill health is abnormal and unnatural. The living body is **always**, under **all** conditions, striving for the very highest level of health for itself that is possible. You can tap into the intelligence of the Universe and unleash its powerful healing potential to ensure for yourself a life dominated by energy and well-being. The trick is to learn how to get out of the body's way and allow it to heal itself of any problem that may develop, which it can and **will** do with a higher degree of effectiveness than anything else in existence. Unfortunately, having never been educated about how to do this, we instead, all too frequently, unknowingly thwart the body's natural tendency to fix itself.

This book is going to change all that for you. It is going to take you on a journey of discovery. Perhaps for the first time in your life you will learn aspects about your own wondrous body that you never knew before—how it works and how profoundly every aspect of your life that concerns your well-being is affected by the manner in which it is treated.

What I would ask you to do, to the best of your ability, is to clear your mind of everything you have ever heard about pain; about Fibromyalgia, Lupus, Arthritis, and Chronic Fatigue Syndrome. Don't read what you are about to read with any preconceived ideas. Pretend that you have never heard a word about them, and allow your common sense, reason, sense of logic, and instincts to be your guide. See if what you read resonates and rings true deep inside of you in a way that tells you in no uncertain terms that you're on to something that can help you.

Over time, people have been convinced that achieving a high energy state of pain-free well-being is complicated or dependent upon luck, "good genes," or some other factor that is out of the individual's hands. The reality is that our actions determine whether or not we will live healthfully or in dis-ease. Life is such that we always have choices. It is the sum total of those choices that determines what our life will be like. Step by step you will learn what pain truly is— what causes it, what purpose it serves, how to remove it, and how to prevent its return. By the end of the book you will know what Fibromyalgia, Lupus, Arthritis, and Chronic Fatigue Syndrome are and exactly what to do to avoid them. And as an added plus you will know that accomplishing that goal is entirely in your power.

CHAPTER ONE

HOPE SPRINGS ETERNAL

It's probably a safe bet to say that on the list of most desired wishes, health is right up there on the very top of the list. Even above tremendous wealth. After all, what use is a lot of money if you're too sick to enjoy it? And if money could bring health, there would be no sick rich people.

You know, it's one thing to develop some painful condition which is diagnosed, explained, and remedied by a specific, time-tested course of action that removes the ailment. It's never any fun being sick, whether it's something minor or major. But at least there's the satisfaction of knowing what it was that made you sick and what was required to recover. You take the proper steps not to repeat what brought on the malady in the first place and move on with your life.

It's an entirely different scenario when things aren't so clear-cut, isn't it? Developing a painful and debilitating condition and being told that "no one knows" the cause and there's really nothing to be done except to deaden the symptoms with an array of drugs and accept that it's something that has to be lived with is depressing and devoid of hope. In other words, a bummer of the first order.

It never ceases to amaze and amuse me when members of the medical profession authoritatively declare that "no one knows" the cause of a certain malady merely because **they** don't know. It's so arrogant. And it is also patently untrue. Just because **they** don't know, it doesn't mean that **no one** knows. But because the medical profession is the dominant health care system in the world, people accept at face value that they know what they're talking about—even when they don't.

It may appear that I'm looking for any opportunity to slam the medical profession, but that's not what this is about. The fact is, numerous disciplines exist in the health-care profession. Not one, but many. There's Medicine, Natural Hygiene, Chiropractic, Osteopathy, Naturopathy, Homeopathy, Acupuncture and Acupressure, Hydrotherapy, Neuromuscular therapy,

Craniosacral therapy, Reflexology, and others. I'm not making a value judgment about which are worthy of attention and which are not. The plain truth is, all exist, all have practitioners that believe wholeheartedly in their particular field of choice, all have something of value to offer, and all can point to successes in people that have utilized the principles of each modality.

The nature of knowledge, be it in the healing arts or any other field of endeavor, is that what is known is but a mere pittance compared to what is not known. All knowledge combined can be compared to a single grain of sand on a vast stretch of beach which represents what is yet to be learned. Thank goodness. Imagine what a bore life would be if everything there was to know was already known. Not a scrap of new information would ever be discovered again. Part of what makes life the interesting journey it is, is not knowing at what point some exciting new bit of information will be discovered in the great unknown.

That being the case, is it not the absolute height of absurdity for members of one group of practitioners, in any profession, be it health care, astronomy, politics, or education, to declare that they have all the answers to questions in their field, and if they don't, no one does?

Well, that is precisely the situation as it exists today in the arena of health care. Above, I listed 12 different disciplines involved in health care, yet one has set itself up as the final arbiter in all questions regarding health and ill health.

Back at the beginning of the 20th century, men with tremendous wealth and power, the Rockefellers and Carnegies, were able to foresee the astronomical profits to be made in the pharmaceutical industry. Under their avaricious direction, colleges that were willing to push drug therapy were given funding and remained open. Those colleges that wanted to focus on other methods that did not depend on drugs were deprived of funding, and they closed.[13] So under those circumstances the drug dominated medical profession became the dominant health care system, and to this day it dominates the landscape in all matters pertaining to health care—to the point where medical doctors sit in judgment of the validity and worthiness of all other modalities, even ones they've never even studied.

Imagine that occurring in any other field. Take law, for example. If you were injured on the job and decided to file a lawsuit, would you seek help from an attorney specializing in real estate law or corporate law? Would you seek the help of a divorce attorney? No, you would seek the help of an attorney specializing in personal injury law. Even if you were to go to a real estate or divorce attorney, s/he would, in all likelihood, direct you to the services of an attorney whose expertise is in personal injury.

A medical doctor acknowledging that s/he is stumped and ill-equipped to explain why someone is sick and then recommending someone in another branch in the healing community is as rare as a Charlton Heston poster demanding gun control. More often than not s/he will merely state that the cause of the problem is unknown and prescribe drugs in an attempt to lessen the symptoms.

I am in no way suggesting that people not seek the services of the medical profession when appropriate. My point is that medical doctors, just like practitioners in other disciplines, have limited and specific areas of expertise, and it is in those areas they should be consulted. Here's what medical doctors are trained in and where they excel: diagnosis, trauma, emergencies, and surgery. What they are **not** trained in and the area in which they are **not proficient** is in explaining and removing long-term, chronic illness.

If you had a compound fracture of the leg or a gaping wound or a diseased organ that had to be removed or a heart attack, I would not recommend you see a Natural Hygienist. I would suggest that you hotfoot it to a medical doctor. By the same token, if you wanted to learn how to eat in order to optimize your health, or you wanted to know how to lose weight or how to remove pain without the use of toxic drugs or wanted an explanation for **why** you are suffering from health problems, not the least of which is Fibromyalgia,

Lupus, Arthritis, or Chronic Fatigue Syndrome, then I would most definitely suggest that you seek the help of a Natural Hygienist who has studied those very things. That way you could learn the **underlying reasons** why you are not feeling well and remove them, rather than battling the symptoms while the **cause** of the problem is left unchecked.

To bring this discussion of who studies what and who knows what to a close, allow me to share one last nugget of information with you that I think you will agree is most revealing and convincing. As I stated earlier, the foundation stone of Natural Hygiene is that the living body is eminently capable of healing itself of any problem, large or small, when given the opportunity to do so. The study of Natural Hygiene is inseparably intertwined with the study of diet and nutrition. Let's face it; food is a fundamental necessity of life. This is not an issue or even a subject of debate. There may be debate about **what** to eat but all agree that we **must** eat. Stop eating and you die. That's it. It could take up to two months or more, but the unassailable fact of the matter is, we must eat to live.

The two vital and indispensable essentials that we must obtain from food are: nutrients to build, repair, and maintain all of the cells that comprise the body, and a source of energy to carry out the innumerable activities conducted by the body. We humans are eating machines—we are here to eat. We will all, on average, each eat an astounding 70 tons of food over the course of our life. Wow! Seventy tons! Some of us food junkies are trying to exceed that amount but that's another story.

How long you will live, how healthy you will be, how much energy you will have, how much pain you will have to endure, how efficiently your organs will function, how much you will weigh, how well you will feel—**all** are almost entirely dependent upon the quality of the food you eat and, even more important, how well that food is digested and assimilated by your body.

Whether you happen to be aware of it or not, there is not a single malady of the human body, from colds to cancer, that cannot ultimately, to one degree or another, be traced back to how well food was digested and assimilated. That is where everything starts—in the stomach. That is why an understanding of diet and nutrition is central in successfully understanding and overcoming Fibromyalgia, Lupus, Arthritis, and Chronic Fatigue Syndrome.

For the same group of people who are telling you there is no known cause for Fibromyalgia, Lupus, Arthritis, and Chronic Fatigue Syndrome, the study of diet and nutrition has never been a priority. In fact, just the opposite is true. As recently as the late 1970s and early 1980s, medical doctors actually ridiculed—made fun of—people who studied diet and nutrition as a means of preventing or healing ill health and disease. As far as they were concerned it wasn't "real doctorin'."

I remember a specific instance on the Larry King show when a medical doctor actually accused CNN of being irresponsible for interviewing someone who was intimating that cancer could be prevented—even healed—by proper diet. As far as the doctor was concerned, it was absurd to even **suggest** that diet had anything to do with cancer. Of course today it is a well established fact that it is. As a matter of fact, by the time the mid-1990s rolled around, the medical community was attributing up to 40% of all cancers to lifestyle habits such as diet,[14] while some estimates place it at a much higher percentage linking dietary factors to up to 80% of cancer of the bowel, breast and prostate.[15]

As it happens, in April 2003 the *New England Journal of Medicine* reported on a study considered to be the largest and most comprehensive of its kind ever conducted—900,000 people over a 16-year period—which indicated that at least 90,000 cancer deaths a year could be prevented by losing weight.[16]

Considering that it is an irrefutable fact that diet and nutrition play an immense roll in one's health, does it not strike you as odd that approximately **75%**

of the medical schools in the United States **do not require a single class on the subject?**[17] Not one hour. What that means is that a person could go to one of over **90** medical schools and receive a medical degree without ever hearing even one word about something as fundamental and crucial to health as diet and nutrition. Does that seem reasonable to you?

Imagine if you will, that you wanted to learn how to sail a boat around the world. You go to the most comprehensive, highly respected sailing school in existence and you learn all about lines, sheets, different types of sails, winches, the theory of sailing, handling a boat in the water, tacking up and back, and how to duck out of the way of the boom. The only thing left out of the course is navigation and piloting. In other words, you would know how to zip your boat all around in the water and what sails to use in order to do so, but once out on the open ocean you would have no clue about where you were or where you were going. How long do you think you would survive? "But that's too ridiculous to even contemplate," you may be thinking. "It would be insane to teach a course on sailing and leave out how to figure out where you were." No more ridiculous than teaching someone how to be a medical doctor and leaving out diet and nutrition.

You may think I'm going on about this a bit too much. Not so; and for two very important reasons. First, a fact of life is that medical doctors' words are taken as

Gospel. So when they say "no one knows the cause" of Fibromyalgia, Lupus, Arthritis, and Chronic Fatigue Syndrome, people believe it and lose hope, even though the medical doctors never studied the very factors that enable others to explain what the people who "don't know" can't explain. I have studied diet and nutrition for 35 years, yet I have personally been on national TV shows where some medical doctor was called upon to sit in judgment of the worthiness of my work even though s/he had not studied diet and nutrition for even 35 minutes. Do you think that's fair and reasonable?

No greater evidence exists of the vice like stronghold that the medical profession has on our lives than the disclaimers that all health books written by non-medical doctors, including this book, **must** contain. It must state clearly that the advice given is **not** intended to substitute for the advice of the reader's physician and that before making any change the reader must consult his or her physician. Wouldn't taking a book on diet and nutrition written by someone who has studied it for over three decades to a physician for validation who has never studied it at all be the same as insisting that before an artist could sell a painting it must first be taken to a blind person who would decide if the painting was worthy of being sold?

I am taking so much time on this subject because it is at the very heart of what you will need to know about how to free yourself from the clutches of

Fibromyalgia, Lupus, Arthritis, and Chronic Fatigue Syndrome. Your key to success depends upon your fully grasping the point I made about the importance of not only the nature of your diet but also how efficiently food is digested and how effectively it is assimilated and utilized by your body.

Now, upon learning that the way to overcome Fibromyalgia, Lupus, Arthritis, and Chronic Fatigue Syndrome is through dietetic maneuvering, you may be thinking, "Uh-oh, I hope this isn't some whacked out, off-the-wall eating regimen where all I get to eat is sprouts and shredded carrots." You can relax; it isn't. In fact, it in no way becomes a clinical endeavor of calorie counting, portion measuring, and deprivation. You'll be pleased to know that no food groups are eliminated, and you can eat the foods you like. The difference will be in what you eat and at what times and in what combinations.

The actual changes I will be recommending you make in your diet are actually so simple and straightforward that some people have difficulty accepting that measures more elaborate and complicated aren't necessary in order to overcome problems as apparently bewildering as Fibromyalgia, Lupus, Arthritis, and Chronic Fatigue Syndrome.

Much to your immense good fortune, you already have the greatest, most powerful ally in existence to assist you: your own body. That's right; the very body that has been such a source of pain in the past is precisely what is going to rescue you from further suffering. The body is the healer, plain and simple. It's merely a matter of learning how to unleash and direct the unsurpassed healing capabilities that are an inherent part of the living human body. Absolutely everything you will need to know to accomplish this will be revealed to you in detail so you will know exactly how to take charge and control of your health and well-being for the rest of your life.

For now, I want you to feel hopeful, not hopeless, feel encouraged and positive about your prospects for the future. Have faith and know that what you need to feel better exists and is real and is about to become known to you.

CHAPTER TWO

CLOUDS ACROSS THE SUN

If, from your earliest recollection, you were told that trees were called rocks and that horses were called rabbits, it would not be at all strange to hear someone say, "Let's saddle up the rabbits and ride into the woods and sit in the shade of the sycamore rocks." Since it would have been the only way you would have ever heard them described, there would be no reason to think it's strange. Only if you heard them referred to as something other than what you had always heard would it be odd-sounding.

Perhaps not the most perfect analogy, but what you have been told about Fibromyalgia, Lupus, Arthritis, and Chronic Fatigue Syndrome and what can be done about them is no more accurate than describing horses as rabbits and trees as rocks.

Before continuing, I want to take just a moment to point out to you a magical little word that the people who "don't know" depend upon the way a bird depends upon its wings in order to fly. I say it's magical because it at the same time gives the impression that more progress is being made in a given area and more is understood about a given subject than is actually the case, while simultaneously removing all responsibility for an unwanted outcome in case what is said turns out to be incorrect. This word is an integral part of the vocabulary of the people who don't know what they're talking about but want you to think that they do, and without it they would very likely be forced to say nothing at all or actually admit that they don't know.

So what is this little word with such far-reaching implications? *May*. That's it—m-a-y. It may be this or it may be that. Or it may be something else, or it may be nothing at all. You can say that anything **may** be so, but when you do, you are by inference saying that the opposite may also be so. The word **may** (and its variations, *maybe, might, can, could, possibly,* and *perhaps*) is used more and relied upon more by the medical/pharmaccutical industry than any other word in the English language.

If you are thinking that I am blowing this out of proportion, you are mistaken. Everyone uses the word **may**, including me: "You may want to think about initiating an exercise routine." But it can also be used to recommend something harmful or even deadly: "This drug may help your high blood pressure." Drugs **always** have the potential of harm because they one and all have negative side effects. There is no way of knowing whom they will help, and whom they will hurt. That is why you will **never** be told by your physician that a certain drug **will** bring about a certain result, only that it **may**.

I am an article collector. I've been cutting articles out of newspapers and magazines for 30 years. I like to use them as a teaching tool because, unlike scientific journals, they are accessible and easy to read. More people look at newspapers or magazines as often as daily, whereas those same people rarely have an occasion or a desire to read a scientific journal. They're written in obscure, unrecognizable jargon, so it's a lot easier to let a journalist glean what is useful information from them and put them in a newspaper or magazine article. I have boxes and boxes of these articles all over my home.

Something that I used to do regularly was, every time I saw a headline pertaining to some aspect of health or ill health that had the word **may** in it, I clipped it out, highlighted the word **may** in florescent yellow, and kept them in separate boxes. I had to stop because I had so many. They were taking up too much space. I threw most of them out, but I kept one box full. As I was writing this section I put my hand into the box and pulled out a half dozen at random. Here they are: ANTIBIOTICS MAY CUT HEART ATTACK RISK;[18] DRUG MAY HOLD CLUE FOR CANCER;[19] CANCER DRUG MAY HELP REDUCE HEART ILLS;[20] BLOOD TEST MAY HELP DETECT CANCERS EARLY;[21] GENE THERAPY MAY HELP BATTLE HEART DIS-EASE;[22] COW-CELL IMPLANTS MAY HELP EASE PAIN.[23] I could fill this book with more of the same.

I have found that many people, perhaps most, will read a headline but not the entire article, or they will read the headline and the first few paragraphs but not the entire article, so at first glance it **may** appear that good progress is being made or at least that researchers are on the right track. But almost without fail, somewhere in the article under the big, splashy headlines you will find the inevitable disclaimer. They go something like this: "Researchers warn us not to expect it (the drug that **may** help) anytime soon." "It **may** be ten years before the product is actually available." "Tests were on mice and **may** not be applicable to humans." "A great deal more research is necessary before there will be a marketable product." "Scientists hope a product will be ready sometime in the future."

It's all speculation and guesswork, and that's all it is. All manner of outlandish speculation is within the realm of possibility as long as it is preceeded by the word **may**. It's all designed to lull you into a false sense of security. I could tell you that my cat **may** learn how to do the dishes, and it's true, she may, but knowing my cat, I doubt it. But she may!

If you will start to pay attention to how often the word **may** is used, not only in articles but also in news reports on the radio or TV, you will be amazed. People don't notice it until it's pointed out to them, but once it is, it seems like a news item on some aspect of health care is rarely complete without the use of the word may. I brought the subject up in the first place because whatever you have been told about what Fibromyalgia, Lupus, Arthritis and Chronic Fatigue Syndrome are, what causes them, and what can be done about them has most assuredly relied heavily upon the word *may*.

Let's take a quick look at what you've been told about Fibromyalgia, Lupus, Arthritis, and Chronic Fatigue Syndrome, and then follow it with the nonfiction version. First, Fibromyalgia, clinically referred to as Primary Fibromyalgia Syndrome (PFS) or Myofascial Pain Syndrome (MPS). Take special note that Fibromyalgia is classified as a syndrome. The word *syndrome* is used to describe a group of symptoms for which there is no explanation. That certainly well describes Fibromyalgia and is precisely why the people who "don't know" classify it as such.

The word *Fibromyalgia* is made up of two words—*fibro*, meaning associated with the body's *connective tissue* fibers, and *myalgia*, which indicates muscle pain. It's startling how few people are familiar with the vital and indispensable role of connective tissue in the body. I cannot think of a single activity of the living body that does not in some way interact with some form of connective tissue. Some connective tissue is exceedingly thin, nearly translucent as cellophane while other connective tissue is thicker and denser. It forms the framework upon which all other body tissues are assembled. Connective tissue is remarkably resilient as it holds all the body parts together, supports organs, transports nutrients to the cells, and gives shape to and supports the body's musculature and skeleton. Bones are a type of mineralized connective tissue; even blood is considered to be a type of connective tissue. All blood vessels are embedded in connective tissue. All throughout the length and breadth of the body, connective tissue is binding, supporting, shaping, protecting, defending, repairing, and nurturing body tissues and cells. And of course connective tissue is an integral component of all muscles.

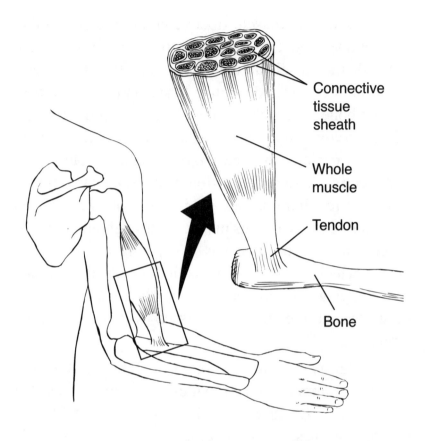

Connective tissue sheath

Whole muscle

Tendon

Bone

If you were to see a cross section of a muscle, you would see what looks like spaghetti strands of fiber, each one wrapped in connective tissue. Bundles of those spaghetti-like fibers are in turn wrapped in connective tissue, and then the entire muscle is sheathed in more connective tissue. So the connective tissue runs in, around, and through the muscle, basically permeating it. The muscle fibers end, but the connective tissue does not. The connective tissue from inside and outside the muscle all comes together, then becomes a tendon of fibrous connective tissue and attaches itself to the bone. Muscles are not attached directly to bone. The *tendons*, made up of connective tissue, actually connect muscles to bone. *Ligaments*, also made up of connective tissue of a different consistency, connect muscles to other muscles and bones to other bones and also suspend the organs in place. Throughout the body, connective tissue connects everything to everything else, which is why it is called connective tissue. Fibromyalgia is, therefore, a condition affecting the muscles and the connective tissue associated with the muscles.

As far as what the symptoms of Fibromyalgia are, they are numerous and widespread throughout the body wherever there are muscles. Most notably are pain, achy-ness, and tenderness localized to specific small zones of the body referred to as "tender points," which are particularly sensitive to touch. In extreme cases, severe, disabling pain occurs with the slightest movement. Being hugged, sneezing, or even going over a bump in the road in a car can be extremely painful. Accompanying this pain is poor sleep, enlarged, tender glands, persistent fatigue, stress, anxiety, and irritability. It ain't fun, that's for darn sure.

Regarding the cause of Fibromyalgia, we already

know that the conventional medical position is that it's a mystery—"no one knows." In order not to appear completely impotent in the face of such a debilitating condition, medical doctors have flung the door of speculation wide open. Of course the most well-worn and often used bugaboo and scapegoat of all time is thrown into the mix: the virus. Yes, it "may" be a viral infection. Or it "may" be a remote bacterial infection. Most people have absolutely no idea in the world what a virus or any other microscopic organism is other than what they have been told by the folks who have no answers to your questions and who want to take the pressure off themselves. Anytime medical people are stumped, they always seem to fall back on the possibility that it "may" be a virus or some other unseen entity at work. Who's to say otherwise? And, hey, it may *not* be a virus.

Other speculative guesses about what **might** cause or exacerbate the condition associated with stress, tension, anxiety, and depression exist, but that's all it is, guesswork based on haphazard circumstances. There is however, **one** factor that is known to amplify the symptoms of Fibromyalgia: being told by your physician that it's "all in your head."

Even though Fibromyalgia was first described in the early 1800s and officially recognized by the American Medical Association as a true major cause of disability in 1987, still some medical doctors refuse to acknowledge that it even exists. Can you imagine

being in unrelenting pain day and night only to have
your doctor suggest that it's probably some psycholog-
ical disturbance that's all in your head as s/he sends
you home with a prescription for Prozac or some other
anti-depressant? Yeah, that would stress **me** out and
cause anxiety and depression. No doubt.

The typical treatment for Fibromyalgia is a journey
through a dangerous minefield of guesswork and trial
and error. Of course numerous measures exist involving all manner of body work, gentle massage, biofeed-
back, acupuncture and acupressure, local applications
of heat, stretching, and exercises, but the standard,
knee-jerk approach to Fibromyalgia is a dizzying array
of drugs. Looking over the list of the dozens of different powerful, sometimes devastating drugs is a daunt-
ing and frightening prospect. Drugs are prescribed to
promote sleep, to relax muscles, many different ones
for the pain that occurs in numerous sites throughout
the body, for fatigue, for migraines, for irritable bowel,
for digestive irregularities, anti-anxiety drugs, anti-
depressants, and anti-inflammatories (even though
Fibromyalgia is not considered to be an inflammatory
condition). There's Elavil, Inderal, Paxil, Prozac,
Tagamet, Zantac, Xanax, and Zoloft, to name but a
few of the more well-known ones.

You should be aware of two extremely important
aspects of this frenzy of drugging. First, the toxic
nature of some of these drugs can have some disas-

trous side effects. Looking over the possible adverse effects is like reading a horror story. They are too numerous to list; literally dozens and dozens. Every part of the body can be negatively affected, including the heart, kidneys, liver, and skin. They can cause headaches, stomachaches, nausea, vomiting, diarrhea, digestive disorders, blood disorders, and immune disorders. The list goes on and on interminably, including in some instances death!

Sometimes a drug for one symptom actually has a side effect of one of the other symptoms you're trying to relieve. They further toxify the body, making progress in overcoming the original problem of Fibromyalgia even more difficult. Some of the drugs, such as Lidocaine and Procaine, are injected directly into areas of particular discomfort. The attitude is, since nothing is actually known about it and nothing can be done to eliminate it we might as well see if we can figure out how to help patients cope with it.

Second, and equally disturbing, is that not **one** of these drugs in any way, shape, or form does **anything** whatsoever to overcome Fibromyalgia. Nothing! These drugs have one purpose and one purpose only, and that is to lessen the effects of the symptoms sufficiently so the patient can get on with some semblance of life as s/he copes with the disease. And since there is no way to tell which drugs will help and which ones will hurt and there exists no technology to determine what effect different drugs in the body at the same time will produce, the entire process of finding the correct drugs is by trial and error. "This one **may** work; let's **try** it. If it doesn't, we'll **try** another, and **maybe** it will work. Or we **can try** a combination and see if it works or **try** another combination if it doesn't."

The idea is to finally stumble across a group of drugs that manages to find that fine line that reduces the symptoms without further harming or killing the patient. Plus, as a final message of hopelessness to the patient and an added acknowledgement of the medical profession's bewilderment on the subject, some of the drugs are recommended to be taken indefinitely. In other words, for the rest of one's life, with the constant monitoring of side effects. Such is the state of affairs regarding the understanding and treatment of Fibromyalgia according to the medical profession.

The two classifications of Lupus are *discoid* and *systemic*. Discoid Lupus is a disorder that confines itself to the skin. This book addresses systemic Lupus, the more common type, because of its similarities to Fibromyalgia. Not that what you are about to learn will not also help relieve discoid Lupus; it will, but it is systemic Lupus I am referring to whenever I use the term *Lupus* within these pages.

Lupus is a disorder of.....the connective tissue! I have linked Fibromyalgia and Lupus together throughout because they are the same disorder. Now I know there are those who will say that they are not the same thing, that they are separate conditions, and in certain specific areas that's true. Lupus is classified as an inflammatory condition; Fibromyalgia is not. Fibromyalgia affects primarily the connective tissue inside muscles whereas Lupus is primarily in the ligaments, tendons, and around the organs. But in the broadest sense they are the same. Both are problems associated with connective tissue.

Everything you have read on the last few pages on Fibromyalgia is also true about Lupus. Both have causes that are supposedly unknown. Both **may** be caused by a virus. Both are extremely painful. Both have similar symptoms of pain, extreme fatigue and malaise, and swollen and tender lymph glands, and both cause depression, anxiety, tension and stress, poor sleep, and digestive problems. And it goes without saying that both are treated with a wide variety of drugs that are administered in the same hit-or-miss fashion. They are essentially the same problem, simply manifesting in slightly different areas of the body. It's no accident that 55% of people diagnosed with Lupus are also diagnosed with Fibromyalgia.[24]

Whenever you see "itis" at the end of a word, it means "inflammation of." So appendicitis is an inflammation of the appendix, dermatitis is an inflammation of the skin, and so on. Enteritis is an inflammation of the intestines. Colitis is an inflammation of the colon. That means a person can have an inflammation of the small intestines, and if that inflammation moves one quarter of an inch into the colon, it is given the different name of colitis. They're not different conditions; they're the result of the same problem. So it is with Fibromyalgia and Lupus. In both, the connective tissue is in distress. So, yes, if pain exists in the connective tissue of a muscle it could be called Fibromyalgia, and if the pain is in the connective tissue of an adjoining tendon or ligament to that muscle, it could be called Lupus, but for the purpose of this book I am talking about how to overcome problems associated with the connective tissue anywhere in the body. That certainly includes Fibromyalgia and Lupus.

Now, as to Arthritis, the number one cause of disability in the United States.[25] The literal meaning of the word Arthritis is *joint inflammation* and it is a painful condition for approximately one in three adults or roughly 70 million people in the U.S. alone![26] Some of you may be wondering, if this is a book about relieving ailments associated with connective tissue in the body, why is Arthritis included? That's easy—Arthritis is a disorder of the connective tissue! Don't worry if this comes as a revelation to you; it puts you into a rather large majority.

The human skeletal system is an intricate web of bones, some large some tiny, that is a marvel of creation and a wonder to behold as it supports and gives shape to the body allowing it to stand upright and basically move in any direction desired. There are 206 bones in the body and every one of them except one in the neck (hyoid bone) forms an attachment with another bone. The point at which that attachment is made is called a *joint*. If not for these joints the skeleton would be stiff and immovable instead of being able to move with such fluid flexibility.

With hundreds of joints in the body there are **over 100** diagnosable ailments related to Arthritis accounting for the 70 million people who have to deal with joint pain every day. Of the 100 ailments of the joints, far and away the two most common forms of Arthritis are *Osteoarthritis* and *Rheumatoid Arthritis*.

The connective tissue associated with Osteoarthritis is called *cartilage*, a thick, tough, rubbery tissue that supports and cushions the skeleton acting as a shock absorber between bones. It is smooth and slick so the bones can move easily when they come into contact with one another. At the point in a joint where the ends of two bones come into contact, *articular cartilage* help the bones glide easily past each other providing a near frictionless and wear resistant surface for joint movement.

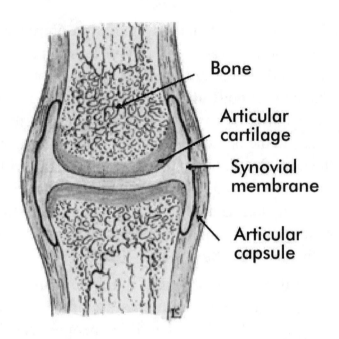

Bone

Articular
cartilage

Synovial
membrane

Articular
capsule

Osteoarthritis, or degenerative joint disease, commonly referred to as the "wear and tear" type of Arthritis is the most common form of all. It occurs when the articular cartilage breaks down and wears away. This allows the bones to grind together, causing pain, swelling, and loss of motion in the joint. Due to the constant friction, the body produces new bone growth called ***bone spurs*** which grow on the edges of the joint. Little bits of bone or even cartilage can break off and float inside the joint space causing even more pain and damage. Over time these spurs can lead to the joint fusing together, severely restricting movement and causing the knobby, misshapen appearance that is sometimes seen in the hands.

If a building is destroyed by fire, investigators may discover that some bad wiring was the cause of the fire and if the building had been properly wired the fire could have been avoided. This is the relationship that Osteoarthritis has to Rheumatoid Arthritis. Although Osteoarthritis can be caused by other means such as an injury, the vast majority of cases are the result of Rheumatoid Arthritis. In fact it would be accurate to say that in most cases Osteoarthritis is the end result of Rheumatoid Arthritis gone to the extreme.

The connective tissue associated with Rheumatoid Arthritis is called the *synovium*. Although amazingly thin, the *synovial membrane* is astonishingly resilient.

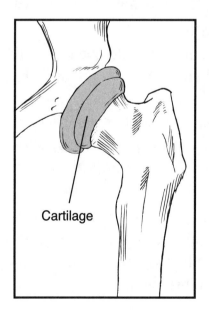

Cartilage

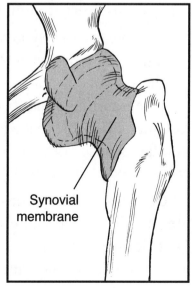

Synovial membrane

It completely surrounds, encases, protects, and nourishes the joints and the cartilage. It does this by determining what can pass into the joint cavity and what cannot, and by producing *synovial fluid*, a clear, sticky substance that provides lubrication and nutrition for the joint.

When the synovium becomes inflamed, otherwise compromised or lost altogether, that is when all the mischief starts. The joint and the cartilage are left completely unprotected. It is then only a matter of time before the cartilage and then the bone begins to deteriorate. And that is how Rheumatoid Arthritis leads to Osteoarthritis. It also explains why the improvement and recovery rate amongst those dealing with Rheumatoid Arthritis far exceed that of those dealing with Osteoarthritis when the recommendations set forth in this book are utilized.

As long as the synovium is intact, even if it is inflamed or otherwise distressed, it can still be repaired when the proper steps are taken. However once the cartilage has been irreparably damaged or lost altogether, due to the loss of the protective synovium, the chances of recovery for Osteoarthritis sufferers is greatly diminished.

Concerning how Chronic Fatigue Syndrome figures into the equation, the connection is a striking one. First, let's review the prevailing opinion of the medical community. As with Fibromyalgia, Lupus, and

Arthritis, the cause is supposedly unknown—"no one knows." As with Fibromyalgia, Lupus, and Arthritis, researchers **suspect** that it might, maybe, may, could, perhaps, possibly be the result of a virus. There's a surprise. As with Fibromyalgia, Lupus, and Arthritis, the symptoms are similar. Although one of the symptoms of Fibromyalgia, Lupus, and Arthritis is fatigue and malaise, with Chronic Fatigue Syndrome the most notable symptom is an overwhelming fatigue, whereas the most notable symptom of Fibromyalgia, Lupus, and Arthritis is pain. Pain is also a symptom of Chronic Fatigue Syndrome and can be experienced as headaches and joint pain. As with Fibromyalgia and Lupus, Chronic Fatigue Syndrome causes muscle weakness, swollen, tender glands, sleep disturbances, irritability and depression. And last, the treatment is— you guessed it—experimental drugs in the hope that one or more "**may**" lessen symptoms.

The similarities between Chronic Fatigue Syndrome and Fibromyalgia bear such a striking resemblance to each other that some doctors assume that Fibromyalgia and Chronic Fatigue Syndrome are the same. Many people diagnosed with Chronic Fatigue Syndrome actually have Fibromyalgia. As you progress through the book, you will become increasingly aware of the way in which Chronic Fatigue Syndrome impacts Fibromyalgia, Lupus, and Arthritis, and how it is in turn impacted by them.

If a person were to go to the doctor in pain and the cause was not something that was easily diagnosed, like Arthritis, there's a pretty good chance that it would be diagnosed as Fibromyalgia, Lupus, or Chronic Fatigue Syndrome, as they have become "catch-alls" for pain and weakness in the body that has no immediately recognizable cause.

I of necessity have to address the most ridiculously absurd notion associated with Fibromyalgia, Lupus, Arthritis, and Chronic Fatigue Syndrome that I have ever encountered. Frankly, I'm dumbfounded that I even have to take the time to deal with it but as it happens, stunningly, it is at the very heart of the medical community's belief system on the subject, enjoying the greatest unanimity amongst medical doctors. I am talking about the fact that Fibromyalgia, Lupus, Arthritis, and Chronic Fatigue Syndrome are all considered to be what is referred to as *autoimmune* diseases.

An autoimmune disease is allegedly when the immune system goes haywire and causes illness by mistakenly attacking the body's own healthy cells, organs, or tissues that are essential for good health. The body's immune system becomes misdirected, attacking the very organs it was designed to protect. The theory is that the immune system loses its ability to recognize some tissue or system within the body as "self" and targets and attacks it as if it were foreign.

Supposedly there is a varied group of more than 80 serious, chronic illnesses that involve almost every human organ system that are considered to be autoimmune diseases. This is medical science fiction at its very worst. I feel like I am in the position of having to seriously prove that there is no tooth fairy or that the moon is not made of green cheese.

In the simplest possible lay terms it goes something like this: Anything in the body that does not belong, does not support the well-being of the body, or is harmful, is called an **antigen**. The immune system produces **antibodies** to search out, destroy, and remove antigens as quickly and efficiently as possible. An example of antibodies that perform this vital function are **White Blood Cells** (leukocytes) such as **Lymphocytes** which are wandering connective tissue cells that go after antigens; and they know what they're doing!

We are being told, and are expected to believe, that these powerful and highly capable antibodies show up at trouble spots in the body and "something" causes them to freak out and start to attack the very cells they are there to protect. What the something is that has the power to pull off such a formidable feat has yet to be determined but the number one "suspected" villain is none other than our friend....the virus! Other "possible" agents that are also under suspicion are bacteria, fungus, germs, and/or genetic, environmental, hereditary,

or hormonal factors. But the virus is the favorite suspect of all at which the finger of blame is pointed.

As the story goes, the antibodies are somehow
tricked, which cause them to attack healthy cells and
cause inflammation which in turn develops into full
blown disease. Has a virus, or bacteria, or any other
microscopic, malevolent beastie **ever** been located,
isolated, pinned down, or even once **seen**? Never! Not
once, not ever, not even close. Nothing! Decades have
passed searching for some phantom bug with bad
intentions to blame our problems on with zero results.
Nothing has ever been found, but the rationale is that
something has to be there otherwise why would the
antibodies show up in the first place. I will answer this
question for you shortly with the nonfiction version.

In some futile attempt to save face or avoid embar-
rassment at not being able to explain why more than
100 million people suffer pain with no reasonable
answer as to why, members of the medical community, without so much as a single scrap of evidence, have
come up with this outlandish and bizarre fairy tale that
makes absolutely no sense, is completely illogical, is
pure speculation and nothing more, is impossible to
prove and never has been proven; nor will it because
there **is** no phantom bug.

The infinite intelligence that so exquisitely governs
the universe and everything in it, including the activi-

ties of the human body, with a precision and exactness that is utterly incomprehensible to us, is indescribably intelligent, powerful, and capable beyond anything we can imagine, not stupid, weak, incapable of protecting itself, and so easily tricked, as the autoimmune theorists would have us believe.

Imagine if you were told that intruders had broken into your home and ransacked the place. You rush home as quickly as possible and when you arrive you find no intruders so in response to the situation you burn your house down. Sound reasonable?

Or when you arrive home the intruders are gone but your children are there surveying the damage. Do you think that there is anything in all of existence that could not only trick you into failing to recognize your **own** children but also capable of causing you to unleash a deadly attack against them? Your own children! That is exactly the premise of the autoimmune theory. You may have unfortunately been misled into accepting this ludicrous, hypothetical tale of fiction based solely on conjecture and nothing more but it is no more accurate than the idea that if you travel too far you will fall off the edge of the planet because it is flat.

A dark, cloudy day with poor visibility is brightened, and one is able to better see, when the clouds move from in front of the sun. All the speculation, theorizing, guesswork, and conjecture that has dominated what you have been told about Fibromyalgia, Lupus, Arthritis, and Chronic Fatigue Syndrome have clouded your ability to see clearly, or to have even a hint of a reasonable understanding of, what these conditions actually are and what causes them, let alone how to intelligently deal with them.

From personal experience I can tell you firsthand what it is like to have something go wrong with your body, watch it deteriorate right before your eyes, and have absolutely no one be able to explain even to the slightest degree what is going on. The overwhelming feeling of helplessness and frustration such a predicament causes tends to take over your life to the point where you can think of little else. I'm not just imagining what it's like to go through such a torment, I lived through this exact situation earlier in my life, and it was the most challenging adversity I have ever had to confront.

I'll share with you the specifics of that challenge a bit later, but for right now I want to tell you that from this point on in the book you are going to learn specific, unambiguous, and definitive information about Fibromyalgia, Lupus, Arthritis, and Chronic Fatigue Syndrome—what they are, what causes them, why they develop in the first place, how to overcome them, and what to do to prevent their reoccurrence. You will find no unsubstantiated theories, no wild speculation that cannot be proven, and no obscure jargon to wade through and try to decipher. It will be straightforward, reasonable, sensible, and logical information that makes sense and is easy to grasp, understand, and implement in your lifestyle so that you can recapture control over your well-being. No longer will it have to be unknown, mysterious circumstances that determine your state of health. You and you alone will be in charge of that.

CHAPTER THREE

CLEANLINESS IS
NEXT TO GODLINESS

There can be no doubt about what the intended message is to the often used statement, "Cleanliness is next to Godliness." Common sense dictates that clean is better than dirty. We eat off of clean dishes, not dirty ones. We regularly wash our clothes because we don't wish to wear them when dirty. We regularly put clean oil in our cars because they won't run well on dirty oil. And, of course, we are ever diligent about keeping our body washed, scrubbed, and clean.

A far cry from, when in 1850 an article entitled "The Abuses of Bathing" in the *Boston Medical and Surgical Journal* declared that, "In our opinion, once a week is often enough to bathe the whole body for luxury and cleanliness. Beyond this we consider bathing to be injurious."[28] How's that for missing the mark? I wonder how many people who are reading this right now would consider not bathing more than once a week.

I could go on and on about the virtues of cleanliness, but why belabor the point. The fact is that everything looks, feels, and functions better, not when dirty, but when clean. And it is right here with cleanliness where your journey of understanding Fibromyalgia, Lupus, Arthritis, and Chronic Fatigue Syndrome begins.

Three basic activities **must** exist and be observable in order for an organism to be declared alive and to continue living. Whether that organism is a one cell amoeba or a full-grown human body, they must exist for life to exist. Here they are:

1. The ability to take in nutrition.

2. The ability to perform some type of metabolism.

3. The ability to eliminate wastes.

Other activities exist that exhibit life such as being able to produce energy, having some means of movement, to propel itself, and the ability to reproduce, but the three mentioned are the primary activities of life. If any one of the three mentioned above is in any way hindered, impeded, or suppressed, the living body or organism will be threatened, and its health will suffer. If any one of the three is stopped, death would ultimately occur. That is how crucial to life the three functions are.

I would like for you to make note of number three up there, the elimination of wastes, because it is the key that unlocks the door to understanding Fibromyalgia, Lupus, Arthritis, and Chronic Fatigue Syndrome. I have been talking about the extreme importance of cleanliness, and it is your body's ability to eliminate wastes that determines the cleanliness of the **inside** of your body. Obviously, a body that is cleansed of wastes and **kept** clean is going to function better and be healthier than a body that is not. It would, therefore, be accurate to say that this book is all about learning what the factors are that either hinder or help the elimination of wastes from the body. You may not now see the importance of or the connection between the elimination of wastes from the body and Fibromyalgia, Lupus, Arthritis, and Chronic Fatigue Syndrome, but you soon will.

Have you ever noticed that whenever the subject of health is being discussed that the discussion invariably focuses on what should or should not be put **into** the body and rarely, if at all, on what should come **out**? The type and quality of food, water, nutrients, supplements—they're all discussed in the context of either being sure to put them in or not put them into the body.

Let me tell you here and now that when your focus switches to what should come out of the body and you start to take the proper and appropriate measures to optimize their removal, that's when the pain free health you desire, which is the natural and normal condition of your body, will become a reality in your life.

Before delving into that for you, I must pay homage to what I said earlier was your greatest ally in your quest for relief from Fibromyalgia, Lupus, Arthritis, and Chronic Fatigue Syndrome: your body. Whenever I write a book or conduct a seminar or even talk to someone one-on-one, I **always**, without fail, put forth my best effort to instill in readers or listeners a newfound reverence for their body that they may not have had. No matter how eloquently I manage to describe the unparalleled magnificence of the workings of the human body, however, I always feel as though I fall short of doing so. It's like trying to describe the indescribable.

Even if I describe with meticulous detail something as astonishing as any one of our senses, say sight or hearing, and I paint an elaborate picture of the astounding and staggering intelligence necessary that allows us to hear and see, it still could never compare to the true miraculousness exhibited by the human body 24 hours a day. That the human body conducts not millions or billions but literally trillions of activities of the most intricate and complex nature every moment, with a precision that puts any computer in existence to shame, and does so for 100 years or more if need be is too mind-boggling even to begin to try to comprehend.

My personal opinion is that no one, no matter how gifted, is able to put into words the true power, ability, and precision of the human body. It's like trying to fully describe God. I love reading books about the nature of God. Whether I am in full agreement with them or not, I enjoy learning about other people's understanding of what God is. There is a word that I invariably come across when reading such books that I rarely see elsewhere. The word is *ineffable*. Webster's Dictionary defines ineffable to be, "Incapable of being expressed in words." Since the human body is universally considered to be God's finest masterpiece, I can see why I never feel as though I have adequately described its true grandeur.

Precisely in this area of having the utmost respect, admiration, and confidence in the unsurpassed capabilities of the human body to protect and heal itself is where the field of medicine and the field of Natural Hygiene find themselves at the polar opposites of each other. From medicine's perspective the human body is a helpless, hapless pawn forever at risk of succumbing to the unrelenting attack of a never ending onslaught of hostile and harmful viruses, germs, bacteria, and other various and sundry enemies hell bent on our destruction.

Hygiene, on the other hand, views the human body as powerful, dynamic, and fully capable of protecting itself and maintaining a consistently high level of good health. So long as the body is provided with the proper care and biological needs, namely a diet that supplies the nutrients and energy required to perform the vital activities of life, ill health will be kept at bay.

Frankly, if the unseen, microbial world truly was as deadly and responsible for our ills as the medical profession suggests they "may" be, the human race would have long ago ceased to exist. Trying to blame the microbial world for our problems is a smoke screen designed to take the pressure off the people who cannot otherwise explain disease, and it is riddled with inconsistencies.

The greatest of these inconsistencies is why, considering that they (viruses, germs, etc.) are present **absolutely everywhere** in numbers too great to even calculate, do some people become sick while others in similar circumstances do not. This glaring inconsistency has long been a real sore spot and source of consternation for those who rely on blaming microbes when no other reasonable diagnosis can be made.

The standard explanation hit upon to explain away this inconsistency is at the very heart of what I hope to impart to you concerning understanding and overcoming Fibromyalgia, Lupus, Arthritis, and Chronic

Fatigue Syndrome. The explanation hinges on one word: *susceptibility*. Who is susceptible and who is not? Surely factors exist that somehow predispose some people to fall victim to the marauding invaders while others are resistant. The **Merck Manual** is the medical profession's bible of some 5,000 possible ailments that can afflict the human body. In the paragraph giving the possible cause of Fibromyalgia it actually states that "a virus or a remote bacteria **may** cause the syndrome to appear in an otherwise predisposed host."[29] But nowhere are the possible factors that would make one person predisposed (susceptible) and another person resistant ever given.

I have been researching and studying the concept of susceptibility as a determining factor in illness long enough to tell you that it always comes down to the condition of what is referred to as the "inner terrain." Guess what the condition of the inner terrain is referring to. **Cleanliness**! Is the inside of the body so silted up and overburdened with wastes that were not eliminated that it serves as the perfect breeding ground for pain, ill health, and disease, or has the inside of the body been sufficiently cleansed of wastes so that ill health and disease cannot gain a stronghold? That is the meaning of susceptibility. That is what determines who is predisposed and who is not. And it will be your every good effort made to ensure that **your** "inner terrain" is clean and thereby functioning at its highest potential that will minimize the possibility of you ever having to deal with Fibromyalgia, Lupus, Arthritis, or Chronic Fatigue Syndrome.

As I stated earlier, along with taking in food and the process of metabolism the body must, of necessity, eliminate wastes. What are these wastes, and where do they come from? As a perfectly normal, totally natural consequence of living, a certain number of wastes, called *toxins*, are generated in the body. This isn't a bad thing; it's part of the grand scheme of things. A certain number of these toxins are always present in everyone's body. No matter how healthy a person is, no matter what the lifestyle, no matter how good the diet, some toxins have to exist.

When you drive your car, waste is released from the exhaust pipe, and a certain amount of sludge and grime builds up in the oil, which is why the oil must be changed periodically. The human body is the same, except that the sludge and grime are in the form of toxins. Problems arise only when more of these toxins are being produced than are being eliminated. And that unwanted and destructive situation can occur as a result of either an insufficient amount of available energy to flush toxins from the body or if the mechanism in charge of removing wastes from the body is too overburdened and bogged down to function effectively. When **both** are the case—insufficient energy

and ineffective flushing—pain and physical ailments are practically guaranteed; it's just a matter of where in the body the problem will occur.

These naturally occurring wastes to which I am referring are generated from two sources. First is from the breaking down, or death, of cells within the body. An astounding number of cells make up the human body. Somewhere in the neighborhood of 100 trillion, and old cells are constantly being replaced by new ones at the impressive rate of over 200 million every **minute**.[30] That means that every day billions upon billions of cells die off, and it is the residue of these spent cells that are toxic and would actually poison the system to death if they were not removed.

The second source of waste in the body, in fact the source that is far greater than that of spent cells, is produced as a result of the process of metabolism—in other words, from the food we eat. And since everyone eats approximately 70 tons of food in a lifetime quite a bit of waste is produced which is also toxic in nature and must be eliminated from the body before it can cause harm or death.

When I talk about the residue produced as a result of metabolism, I am not referring solely to what is left over in the intestines and bowels after what the body needs from it is extracted. It is far more extensive than that. Your entire body is made up of those 100 trillion cells I referred to a moment ago. Your heart, your bones, your skin, your blood, your **connective tissue**—all are comprised of cells. Every last one of these cells is itself a miniature processing plant, taking in fuel, performing tens of thousands of activities, and producing wastes. Every last cell in your body produces a certain amount of waste that must be collected and removed.

So spent cells and the residue of metabolism are constantly, without letup, generating waste—toxic waste that **must** be regularly and efficiently removed from the body before it can cause harm.

What I am about to say next is going to be most provocative for many of those who are reading this. I do not make this statement lightly. I make it as a result of my own 35 years of study, research, and experience and because it is at the very core of why the field of Natural Hygiene is so effective in improving one's overall state of health. Most of the ailments that exist and which are, according to the medical profession, of unknown origin, are the direct result of uneliminated toxins that pollute and poison the system from the inside and cause most of the pain, ill health, and disease that afflict human beings.

Don't get me wrong. I'm not saying that **all** problems of the body are the result of uneliminated waste. After all, one can be poisoned or smoke cigarettes for years or breathe in asbestos or come into contact with environ-mental pollutants that wreak havoc inside the body and on the skin. I know there are variables that come into play and contribute to ill health in ways that **no one** can fully grasp. But unlike the prevailing mindset that declares that numerous causes of ill health exist, most of which are unknown, I am telling you that most, truly **most** of the maladies associated with pain, ill health, and disease are the result of the uneliminated, poisonous wastes that accumulate in the body over the years.

I decided to write this book specifically because Fibromyalgia, Lupus, Arthritis, and Chronic Fatigue Syndrome are textbook examples of exactly what I am talking about. For years I have used these supposedly four different ailments with no known cause as the classic example of what can happen when one lives a lifestyle that encourages the buildup of waste in the body versus one who actively and consciously supports the body's own efforts to rid itself of waste.

I have long been a huge fan of the analogy as one of the best teaching tools available. In a previous book I was talking about this very subject and came up with what I think is the perfect analogy to make my point. Rather than trying to invent another equally effective analogy, I think I will borrow that one from myself. Sadly, this analogy became a reality in Asia at the end of 2004.

Visualize if you will, a coastal community at the foot of a mountain, with houses all along the coast, some inland, and some near the base of the mountain. If offshore, deep in the ocean, an earthquake occurs, it will send a tidal surge of water crashing right into our little coastal community. The water will destroy a certain number of houses. The earthquake sends boulders from the mountain crashing down on some other houses. And fires started by snapping electrical lines destroy yet other houses. So here we have houses destroyed by water, falling rocks, and fire. Now fire and water are about as different as two things can be. And boulders are like neither. The houses are destroyed by three different means. But all three had the same **cause**! If not for the earthquake, there would be no tidal wave, no falling boulders, and no fires.

What I am telling you is that uneliminated toxins are the cause of Fibromyalgia, Lupus, Arthritis, and Chronic Fatigue Syndrome. They may **appear** to be separate and distinct problems, just as it would appear to someone that the houses in the analogy were destroyed by three different means if s/he was not aware of the earthquake, which was the true cause.

Here's what happens inside the body when wastes, for whatever reason, are not regularly eliminated: Remember earlier when I pointed out that wastes are not eliminated because there's not enough energy and the system in charge of waste removal is too overburdened to function properly? As a result, the wastes settle into, or are stored, in the tissues of the body for removal at some future date when there **is** sufficient energy and the system for the removal of wastes **is** functioning effectively. The storing of these toxins is where all the mischief starts. It is **where** the toxins are stored that determines what particular ailment will develop and what name it will be given.

A dozen people with the **exact same** negative lifestyle habits will not necessarily develop similar problems. You see, everyone has his or her own weakest link. So, yes, it's possible that more than one person out of the 12 will develop the same problem, but it's not likely. Obviously, when the numbers go up and we're talking about millions of people, you will start to see the same problem occur more frequently. That's part of the wonder and mystery of the human body. Except for certain genetic tendencies, **no one** can figure out or predict exactly how each individual body will react to the effects of uneliminated waste. So with one person the waste may settle in the pancreas and cause diabetes. In another it may settle in the arteries and cause heart disease. In another it may settle in an organ and disrupt its ability to function. In another it may settle in the lining of the intestines and cause irritable bowel, colitis, or Crohns disease. And in others it may **settle in the connective tissue and cause Fibromyalgia, Lupus, or Arthritis.**

I have seen firsthand the lessening of pain and the increase in energy in people with Fibromyalgia,

Lupus, Arthritis, and Chronic Fatigue Syndrome who have been willing to make the dietary changes necessary to reverse these conditions. And that is why this book is all about how to remove accumulated toxins from the body and how to eat in such a manner in the future so as to produce the lowest number of toxins possible.

You know that feeling you have right after you've had your car washed? You pull out of the car wash, and it seems as though the car is actually running better. It doesn't matter if the fender is dented or the paint job is faded. There's just something about driving a freshly washed car that feels good. You know what I'm talking about, don't you? Let me ask you another question. Do you think that a car **could** actually run better simply by washing it? We both know the answer, and that answer is: No way. You can spit-shine and polish a car, give it a thorough detailing, wax it, even give it a fresh new paint job, new tires, and new upholstery, but unless the inside of the car receives the same amount of periodic maintenance as the outside, no amount of outer refurbishing or cleansing will have the slightest effect on how the car runs.

When the oil and lubricants are changed, when the gaskets, pumps, hoses, and spark plugs are replaced, when the battery is fully charged—that's the kind of maintenance that must be regularly preformed to ensure a well running car. And it is precisely the same with our body.

Most people, I'm sure, regularly maintain their outer body by showering or bathing every day. They shampoo their hair, clip their nails, and brush their teeth. It's hard to even imagine someone's going weeks, months, or even **years** without performing these basic acts of cleanliness. But you'd be shocked to learn how many people go for **decades** without making even the slightest effort to maintain and cleanse the **inside** of their body. After all, it's the inside of the body that keeps us alive. The outside is just for show.

Most people would cringe at the idea of going to a party with a group of friends with filthy clothing, their hair dirty and disheveled, their teeth gunked up with days' worth of foodstuff, and their body putting off a foul and offensive odor from a lack of bathing. Doesn't sound too appealing, does it? But the same people who may make a disgusted look on their face at such a prospect as that never have even a fleeting thought about what measures they could take to see to it that the same kind of maintenance they are sticklers about for the outside of their body is also provided for the inside of their body. Most people wouldn't **dream** of missing the regularly scheduled maintenance and tune-up of their car but think nothing of depriving their body of the same kind of attention.

Not that what I'm talking about is difficult or complicated or expensive. It's not as though it means taking some funky-tasting concoction that costs hundreds of dollars to clean out the body and remove toxins. No, it is something that the living, intelligent body does for itself as part of an instinctive, ongoing effort to optimize its health by removing waste. The only way the body **won't** perform this vital function of cleansing is if it is somehow prevented from doing so. And that, dear reader, is exactly what millions of people are unwittingly doing. They have never been told of its importance, and, more importantly, they have never been shown how to **get out of the body's way** so it can do what it is fully capable and desirous of doing.

Your body doesn't have to be forced, coerced, or prompted in any way to perform this life-enhancing activity; it only has to be given the opportunity to do so. It is automatic. You don't have to force your eyes to blink. You don't have to force your lungs to inhale after you have exhaled. You don't have to force your stomach to release digestive juices when food enters.

A perfect example of what I am striving to relate to you is what happens when you cut your finger. Even though what takes place when you cut your finger is remarkable and extraordinary, it's something that is taken totally for granted. You know full well a cut finger doesn't mean that all your precious fluids will seep out and you'll die. What you know is that the body will fix it, and fix it, it does. Again, it's not something that you have to force or prompt the body to do; it is something that the body does for itself to protect itself. In fact, except for keeping the wound clean and leaving it alone, nothing has to be consciously done. It's all handled by the supreme intelligence I have praised throughout the book.

First, the body knows to coagulate or thicken the blood so it will stop flowing out. Then it produces a hard casing (scab) that covers and protects the wound while the skin is repaired underneath and joined back together. The hard casing falls off, and as though by magic the wound is healed, and more often than not there's no scar or any trace of where the cut was. **WOW**! That is impressive. The body expertly does all of this for itself no matter what else is going on, no matter what else it has to do.

Even while your body is pumping six quarts of blood through 90,000 miles of blood vessels, while it is maintaining your balance and temperature, while it is turning food into blood, bone, skin, teeth, hair, and organs (an astonishing feat which is beyond what any scientist could possibly do), while it is conducting the numberless tasks of everyday life, it still instantaneously does what is necessary the moment the skin is pierced. And it doesn't matter how tired you are either. You could come home at the end of a long day dead tired and ready to collapse, and if you cut your finger your body will snap into action with the same urgency and efficiency it would if you were just waking up in the morning renewed and refreshed.

You should know that it is with the same urgency and the same efficiency that the body wants to rid itself of waste. It is something that goes on 24 hours a day without letup, because the health, the very **life** of the living body is at stake. Never lose faith in what I refer to as the "dynamics of the living body," which is the natural, instinctive quest for the highest state of health possible. Nothing less is acceptable.

The medical profession's failure to recognize and support the body's own healing capabilities will ultimately go down as one of the greatest blunders in all the history of the healing sciences. It's right up there with bleeding the sick and declaring that cigarette smoking was a "harmless pastime up to 24 cigarettes a day and a pack a day could keep lung cancer away."[31] Drugs actually **suppress** the dynamics of the body, not only **preventing** the healing that would have otherwise taken place if not interfered with and thwarted, but also allowing the original problem to progressively worsen.

Knowing that your body is constantly producing waste as a physiological necessity of life and that the living, intelligent body is constantly striving to eliminate those wastes for its own survival, what do you think the chances are that the Grand Creator of all and everything would **forget** to supply your body with a mechanism to perform the vital function of waste removal? Rest assured that the ineffable intelligence that created and governs all that is, did **not** forget something so crucial to life itself. No way, no how.

If you knew without a doubt that a specific system existed in your body for the express purpose of breaking down and removing waste, thereby dramatically improving your chances of living a long life free of pain, ill health and disease, would you want to know what that system was and what you could do to strengthen and optimize its efforts? It's almost foolish to ask such a question, because who in his or her right mind would **not** want to know?

Such a system does indeed exist in your body, and if you will turn the page I will describe it to you.

CHAPTER FOUR

RUBIES IN THE SAND

Take a moment and picture yourself walking along the shore of a secluded island. You're alone, and you decide to sit down in the sand and take in the beauty of the sky and sea. As you're sitting there letting the warmth of the sun wash over you and listening to the water lap onto the shore, you lean back, and just beneath the sand your fingers feel something cool and hard. You pick it up, and in your hand is a beautiful red ruby glistening in the sun. As you feel around in the sand you discover dozens more precious jewels—diamonds, rubies, emeralds, and sapphires—all beautiful and all yours. I guess it would be pretty safe to say that you would feel mighty fortunate to have discovered such a treasure, would you not?

I would like to help you discover a treasure of even greater worth than a chest full of precious jewels. It's not a treasure of monetary wealth but one of superior physical health. More often than not, people choose uninterrupted good health when asked to choose which they would prefer. Interestingly, you already own the treasure about which I'm speaking—we all do. But, ironically, most people don't have a clue.

We've already learned that the three primary activities of life are the taking in of nutrition, metabolism, and the elimination of the waste produced by metabolism. Hopefully the last chapter was successful in impressing upon you the extreme importance of removing toxin-laden waste from the body before it causes pain, catastrophic damage, or even death.

The supremely intelligent human body which I have been in constant praise of throughout this book has different organs, glands, fluids, and systems that all have very specific functions. It's all very specialized. For example, the cardiovascular system is involved with the circulation of oxygenated blood and is not involved in the digestion of food. Similarly, the digestive system is involved in the digestion of food and is not involved in the circulation of blood. We have the musculoskeletal system, nervous system, reproductive system, and others, all of which have their own specific and particular job to do. They all work in harmony with one another in a highly synergistic way to support the activities and the life of the living body.

The treasure I want to introduce you to is what is referred to as "the body's garbage collector." That's not how it's listed in the index of a physiology book, but that's what it is nonetheless. In physiology books it is called the *lymphatic system*, or lymph system for short. The lymph system is a truly astounding network of glands, nodes, nodules, vessels, and fluid, and its sole job and function is to keep you alive, well, **and free of pain.**

Over the course of the last 20 years, as a result of the term **AIDS** becoming a permanent part of our vocabulary, we have heard with almost monotonous regularity the admonition to do whatever we possibly can to strengthen and boost our immune system. What that advice is in effect saying is strengthen your lymph system, because **the lymph system is the heart and soul of the immune system**. Most everyone has heard references made to leukocytes, lymphocytes, or white blood cells and knows that what are being referred to are the protectors of the body's well-being as was discussed previously. They are on constant alert to seek out and neutralize anything in the body that is not supporting its health and may therefore be a threat.

In terms of whatever health goals we might have, it's hard to imagine anything more important than taking care of our lymph system to the best of our ability. After all, not only is it the nucleus of the immune system but it also is in charge of collecting the waste generated from every last one of the 100 trillion cells, along with all the billions of spent cells, and preparing it for elimination from the body.

The lymph system is not merely a bunch of lymph nodes and glands spread throughout the body. On the contrary, it is unimaginably complex and extensive within the body. In addition to the countless number of nodes and glands, some large, some ever so tiny, the lymph system also includes and makes use of the thymus gland, thoracic duct, spleen, bone marrow, tonsils, appendix, and miles and miles of lymphatic vessels, which contain **three times more lymph fluid than blood**.[32] That last fact alone should be more than enough evidence of the unquestionable importance of the lymph system. All together, with each part making its own contribution, the lymph system constantly filters and purifies the bloodstream, cleansing all the tissues and organs of waste, while regularly produced scavenger cells (lymphocytes, etc.) search out and destroy any harmful material that may enter the body. Whenever you hear anything about the human body's defense mechanism, it is referring to the lymph system, without which life would quickly come to an abrupt halt.

If you could somehow see a close-up view of any part of the inside of the body, you would see, **every-**

where, what would look like intricately woven spider webs covering and surrounding everything. That's the lymph system. You couldn't stick a pin into any part of the inner body without piercing the lymph system. As mentioned earlier, every one of the 100 trillion cells generates a certain amount of waste. The lymph system is right there to immediately pick it up, break it down, and carry it to one of the four channels of elimination: bowels, bladder, lungs, and skin.

You know what the most startling fact of all is regarding the lymph system? The one thing that makes you scratch your head in disbelief? It's how few people have even an inkling of an idea of what the lymph system is or the vital role it plays in acquiring and maintaining good health. It is the ultimate determining factor in the length and quality of life. Good health and all the joys that accompany it is more desired than any other thing. The lymph system is instrumental in achieving that lofty and sought-after goal, but people know practically nothing about it or what it does. What a monumental irony.

If you doubt what I am saying, just start asking people at random if they know what their lymph system is or what it does. It's almost comical as people roll their eyes, scrunch up their face as they search for an answer, and look perplexed, as though you just asked them to spell chrysanthemum—backward! Some people will point to the side of their neck and say something to the effect of, "Yeah, isn't there one right here?" This is the mechanism in their body that determines how long they live and how healthy they will be! It is rare indeed to ask what the lymph system is and have someone answer, "Yeah, it's the body's garbage collector and immune system and keeps us alive and well." I mean it. For your own satisfaction, and fun, start asking people and see for yourself how few of them have even a clue.

If you are one of those people who, until reading this, did not know what the lymph system is, perhaps you can take solace in the fact that even many of the people who you would fully expect to know don't know. I don't want to give the impression that one part of the lymph system is any more important than any other part, because all parts are important. The entire system, with all of the different components, all work together as a cohesive unit to achieve health and well-being for the living body.

I do wish to single out one of the more impressive components of the lymph system and bring it to your attention. It represents the most classic illustration imaginable of the complete and sorrowful misunder-standing of the dynamics of the body in general and the lymph system specifically. In addition to the countless number of lymph glands that are so small they can't be seen, there are many that are quite large and can actual-ly be felt on the side of the neck, under the arm, and where the leg meets the torso. Plus many more relatively large ones are interspersed throughout the body. I want to tell you about not only the largest lymph nodules in the lymph system but also the only part of the amazing lymph system that can actually be seen from the outside of the body by merely opening your mouth and looking in a mirror—the tonsils! Of course many if not most people, including me, cannot see them because they've been yanked out and thrown in the trash.

I could use the space of this entire chapter to describe what a wondrous marvel of creation the tonsils are and what an indispensable role they play in the overall activities of the lymph system and still not fully portray their full worth. There are actually several tonsils. The most common, the ones people think of when they think of tonsils, are on each side of the throat. Then there is a tonsil on the roof of the space above the throat and behind the nose (commonly referred to as adenoids). There are tonsils surrounding the opening of each tube to the ears, a cluster of tonsil tissue at the base of the tongue, and a tonsil in the larynx, or "voice box." These tonsils are all connected by means of lymphatic vessels and form a ring of protection all around the opening of the oral and nasal cavities that provides a defense against bacteria and other potentially harmful materials.

When the lymph system is so overburdened with waste that it can't keep up with its removal, the tonsils fill up, enlarge, and become tender. **This is by design**. This is no haphazard occurrence. It is the intelligent body's way of warning us that something is wrong. The tonsils could not possibly be more strategically placed to perform this vital and life-saving service of warning for us.

Since most of the waste generated in the body is the result of metabolizing the food we eat, what do you suppose the body's message is when the throat practically closes up and it hurts with **every** swallow? Nothing could be more obvious unless our lips suddenly fused together, making it impossible to eat. The unmistakable message is for us to either stop eating or to eat very differently for a while in order to give the lymph system a chance to catch up; which is exactly what would happen if we gave it the chance. If we reduced food intake and drank water and juices and ate very lightly, the toxic level would go down and the tonsils would stop hurting and quickly return to their healthy and proper condition. What do we do instead? We have the tonsils yanked out at the roots and eat a bowl of ice cream to commemorate the occasion.

Until only very recently, the tonsils were considered by the medical profession to be a troublesome and throwaway, nonessential accessory that was more of an inconvenience than anything else. Can you imagine? Can you even begin to fathom the monumental ignorance necessary to suggest that The Master

Designer, The Grand Creator, God, The Intelligence of the Universe, whatever you want to call it, either accidentally or mischievously stuck tonsils in our throat as some kind of cosmic trick or mistake? And at the first opportunity, with the least bit of provocation, they should be torn out? It's too bizarre to even contemplate, and yet that has been the standard procedure for the tonsils for as long as there has been a means of removing them.

I wonder what you would think of this scenario: A person who owns a lot of very expensive jewelry and other valuable belongings and has an extremely elaborate and costly alarm system installed at home to protect against burglary. One night, while that person is asleep, a burglar enters the house and sets off the alarm. The owner of the house, disturbed by the noise, gets up and tears out the alarm so s/he can go back to sleep undisturbed, while the burglar makes off with all the goods. Make sense?

The tonsils are part of the body's alarm system, warning of the impending danger that will occur if the proper steps aren't taken to avert it. Does it make sense to tear out the tonsils (the alarm system) rather than properly caring for the body and giving it a chance to correct the situation? Has your bladder ever been so full that you were actually in pain and all you could think about was relieving yourself? It's probably a safe bet that everyone has experienced that feeling at least once. Is there any possibility whatsoever that you would even **consider** having your bladder surgically removed to deal with the discomfort? Of course not. I know that. Even to say it in jest is beyond absurd, a grotesque idea. It would be removing the bladder for performing the very job it was specifically designed to perform. Preposterous! And yet the tonsils are surgically removed for doing the very job they were specifically designed to perform. Equally preposterous.

The tonsils are not the only essential part of the body's defense mechanism to be treated with ignorance and disdain that borders on contempt. All of which is unwarranted, I might add. The appendix. Here again the medical profession views the appendix as a completely worthless, troublesome inconvenience that exists for the sole purpose of causing pain, grief, and aggravation. Wrong again. I know people who, upon awakening from a surgical operation for something entirely unrelated to the appendix, were told that while the surgeons were in there, they went ahead and removed their appendix for them. Since they were there already, there was no extra charge.

As is the case with the tonsils, the appendix is perfectly and strategically placed at the spot where the small intestine empties into the colon. It is right at the opening of the colon and not anywhere else along the digestive tract or anywhere else in the body because the appendix secretes a substance that breaks down and removes impacted fecal waste from the walls of the colon.

Use your common sense. Doesn't it seem far more logical and reasonable to assume that the tonsils and appendix are integral parts of the wisdom, intelligence, and grandeur of the amazing human body? That **all** parts are essential or else they wouldn't be there in the first place? That the dynamics of the body demand that every part is essential in its own way and they all work in perfect harmony with one another? How many times have you heard someone say, "Human beings are God's finest creation"? I doubt seriously that God's finest creation is littered with unnecessary "extra" parts and imperfections.

The same people who don't give a second thought to removing these vital and valuable organs I have been discussing are the ones who declare that "no one knows" the cause of Fibromyalgia, Lupus, Arthritis, and Chronic Fatigue Syndrome.

Before continuing, I know some of you have had your tonsils or appendix or **both** removed and are thinking, "Uh-oh, I've had it." I'm not going to lie to you and say that it makes no difference if you have those organs intact or not. After what you've just read, certainly you can see that you're better off **with** them than without. But I will tell you that even though your body's defense system has been compromised, you can still, unquestionably, be successful in overcoming Fibromyalgia, Lupus, Arthritis, and Chronic Fatigue Syndrome with the proper care and treatment of your lymph system. I have seen people accomplish that very goal under those very circumstances. All it means is that those who **have** lost one or both of these vital organs will have fewer tools to work with and will therefore have to be particularly diligent in the use of the guidelines I am about to share with you, which are designed to clean and strengthen the lymph system.

What I want to be sure of is that you are heartened and encouraged to learn that your lymph system is tirelessly and impressively endeavoring to remove toxins from all corners of your body—working for your highest health at all times. No vacations, no days off, no breaks. Although there are times when its efforts are more heightened, it is always striving for the highest level of health possible under any and all circumstances. It **must** do this, no matter what. That is why it exists.

In the same way that the body heals a cut finger it also strives to remove toxins. And it stays the course until the job is done. If you fell and cut yourself in 20 places, all would be attended to equally. The body doesn't take the attitude of, "Hey, I'll mend 15 of these cuts, but I'm too busy to handle all 20, I have too much to do as it is." No way. **All** are healed. And even though the body's lymph system may be unwittingly thwarted in its attempt to remove waste (by counterproductive eating and living habits), it never gives up the effort to cleanse the body. It always does the best it can as it waits patiently for obstructions to its effort to be removed.

The human body is incredibly resourceful as it cleverly and skillfully does whatever it has to do in order to protect the vital organs from the toxins that could damage them if not dealt with properly. It not only uses the ordinary means of dealing with toxins, that of gathering them up and breaking them down for removal via the normal channels of elimination (bowels, bladder, lungs, skin), but it also uses certain **extra**ordinary means when the normal channels are overwhelmed.

If it were somehow possible for you to see a video of the entire network of the lymph system in action, you couldn't help but be impressed. Waste from every spot in the body is picked up, broken down, and channeled to the organs of elimination. Throughout the maze of uncountable nodes, nodules, and glands, most of which are too small to see, there are, interspersed throughout, larger glands performing the task of holding and storing waste. That is why sometimes they swell up and are tender. They're full of toxins, which are held there so they won't cause damage to vital organs.

Remember in the beginning of the book when I listed the symptoms of Fibromyalgia, Lupus, Arthritis, and Chronic Fatigue Syndrome? All four had in common swollen, tender glands. That is no coincidence. Sometimes when the workload is heavy and waste is being produced faster than it's being eliminated, a sac is produced to hold waste until the lymph system can catch up. These sacs are called tumors. Most people equate a tumor with cancer, as if they were the same thing. They're not. You would be surprised to know how many tumors come and go in the body without our ever being aware that they were there.

Tumors fill up and empty the same way you fill up and empty the trash can in the kitchen. When they're full they're taken out to the curb in a bag, and a garbage truck comes along and picks them up. When the garbage truck fills up, it empties the load in a landfill and starts over. The same way trash cans are filled and emptied and garbage trucks are filled and emptied, tumors are filled and emptied as well. Many people who feel a lump somewhere in their body freak out, thinking it's cancer, but 12 out of 13 of these lumps are benign.[33] These self-manufactured sacs are only one of the extraordinary means the lymph system uses to keep the toxins they contain from doing damage elsewhere in the body.

Another means by which the body rids the system of toxins when they are in excess of what the normal channels can handle is to expel more of them directly through the skin than usual. Bear in mind that not only is the skin the largest organ of the body but it is also an eliminative organ. As part of the normal, daily process of removing toxins from the body, the skin's four million pores are regularly used. All manner of skin conditions, including the type of Lupus referred to earlier (discoid), inflammation, psoriasis, eczema, staph, shingles, open sores, rashes and pimples, and all the itching, flaking, and irritation that accompany these conditions are far more often than not the result of an overload of toxins that are being pushed out through the skin. In fact, the very steps that you will be taking to overcome Fibromyalgia, Lupus, Arthritis, and Chronic Fatigue Syndrome will also result in much healthier skin.

Yet another **extra**-ordinary means of elimination that the body uses to expel waste that is in excess of what is usual and normal can be seen during what is referred to as a cold. When the level of toxins in the body is such that they are going to cause serious harm, the intelligent body makes use of a cold to dramatically lower the level of toxins quickly by coughing, sneezing, and spitting up phlegm and mucus. An interesting fact that is usually known only to those people who are fortunate enough to still have their tonsils intact is that at the very onset of a cold the tonsils enlarge and become tender, and they stay that way throughout the cold. After the cold has run its course, the tonsils return to normal. Right now some of you who still have your tonsils are saying, "Hey, he's right. My tonsils always swell up and hurt when I have a cold."

Some people's body will use all three of the extraordinary means of elimination I've discussed (tumors, skin, colds); some will use none; and some will use only one or two. As I stated earlier, everyone's body is unique in that regard, and there is no way of knowing whose body will do what. One thing is for certain, and there is no doubt about the fact that if more waste (toxins) is generated in the body than is eliminated, there's going to be trouble. There **has** to be. Those toxins are poisonous, and they have to go.

You know I'm fond of analogies, especially ones involving water or being on the ocean. Here's one to make my point about the results of more toxins being produced than are being removed. Imagine someone alone out on the water in a small boat that sustains damage to the hull bad enough to where quite a bit of water is coming on board. Our lone sailor has no choice but to start bailing water out, or else the boat will capsize. If more water comes in from the breach than s/he is able to bail out, what do you think will ultimately happen? You don't have to have a genius I.Q. to figure that out. The boat will sink!

The lymph system is bailing waste from your body all the time, day and night. As long as it is bailed out at the same rate that it is produced, everything is fine. As soon as the balance tilts in the direction of **less** being removed than is produced, that spells trouble in the short term and in the long term.

Consider the praise that I have taken every opportunity to heap onto the intelligence of the universe that courses through and governs the human body. Truly, I and many other researchers in the life sciences all over the world feel that the true measure of the intelligence and the capability of the human body will never be fully grasped. That being the case, it is absolutely inconceivable that a system as exquisitely designed as the lymph system would not have a built-in warning mechanism to alert us when more waste is being produced than eliminated. After all, it is a life-threatening situation, and the lymph system's reason for being is to protect and conserve life. If there were **not** such a warning mechanism in place and toxins were allowed to continue building in the body unchecked, the result would be a slowly progressing, ever increasing disease state. Over time, minor discomfort would lead to ill health, then sickness, which would lead to more serious disease, then to catastrophic disease, and ultimately to death.

The intelligent body would **not** just sit idly by as it became more and more saturated with toxins without sounding an alarm. **Of course such a warning system exists.** To even suggest that it doesn't would be to suggest that the Grand Creator actually forgot, or was too shortsighted, to supply the super highly sophisticated human body with a system to protect itself and which could be the difference between health and disease and life and death. I don't think so.

I told you earlier that the tonsils are the first line of defense, that they swell up and hurt when the toxic load has surpassed the lymph system's ability to remove it through the normal channels of elimination. But the tonsils are only part of the story. Earlier I was pointing out that we have to regularly change the oil in our cars or it will become so silted up with grime that the car will stop running. Cars have a perfect warning system: a little red light blinks on the dashboard and doesn't stop until whatever is wrong is corrected. Now it would be great if, when we looked in the mirror in the morning, a little red light was flashing right in the middle of our forehead letting us know that our lymph system was being pushed beyond its capacity, but obviously there isn't.

It is so overwhelmingly important that we be alerted as soon as possible to the fact that the lymph system is in distress, overburdened, and in need of some cleansing in order to allow it to bring the toxic level down that the body uses its most reliable, unmistakable, and infallible tool of all to get our attention. Can you figure out what that is? The one tool that cannot possibly be misconstrued and indicates unquestionably that the body is asking for help? Take your time. Don't let me rush you. Think about it for a moment. Give up? It's **pain**! That's what pain **is**. Its purpose is to get your attention. Does it succeed? Does pain get your attention? Is pain something you can easily ignore, or is it something you **can't** ignore? That's the whole idea!

Pain is not some haphazard occurrence that comes and goes for no explainable reason. Nothing in the entirety of our universe just happens. Not a leaf falls from a tree outside the realm of cause and effect. Sometimes the cause of pain is obvious and undeniable. If you stub your toe or smack your finger with a hammer, you're not wondering why you're in pain. It is pain that is not as easily discernable as a stubbed toe or smashed finger that not only opens the door to speculation and guesswork but also causes the kind of frustration that leads to a willingness to **try** to fix it with drugs that actually do more harm than good.

For people such as me, who have made a study of the true cause of pain, ill health and disease, the cause of Fibromyalgia, Lupus, Arthritis, and Chronic Fatigue Syndrome is as obvious as what causes a finger to hurt when it has been hit by a hammer. To state it as simply as I possibly can, **the symptoms of Fibromyalgia, Lupus, Arthritis, and Chronic**

**Fatigue Syndrome are the direct result of unelimi-
nated toxins**. They are in the connective tissue, causing pain. The lymph system has not been able to
remove the toxins because it's overburdened with trying to deal with the overload of the waste in the body
that brought on the problem in the first place.

The only means the body has to alert you to the
predicament that the lymph system is in is to make you
hurt, hoping that you will correct the problem. **Pain
has purpose**. As difficult a concept as it may be for
you to accept, pain has a positive side to the extent that
it is a friendly messenger alerting you to the situation.
I know that if you're in pain every day it's hard to look
at it as a friend, but that doesn't alter the fact that the
pain is trying to warn you about even greater pain and
further suffering if certain changes aren't made. If you
should accidentally put your hand on a hot stove you
would immediately pull your hand away. It would be
the pain you experienced that led you to protect yourself by not leaving your hand on the stove; an obvious
example of pain playing a positive role. The pain associated with Fibromyalgia, Lupus, Arthritis, and
Chronic Fatigue Syndrome will only continue so long
as the cause continues.

I want to be clear about something here. Chronic,
debilitating pain, certainly the kind of pain associated
with Arthritis, Fibromyalgia, Lupus, and Chronic
Fatigue Syndrome, doesn't just happen over night. It

takes a long time; it takes prolonged and sustained neglect of the lymph system's needs to finally result in persistent, unremitting pain. It can, and usually does, take years. But all during the time that it is developing, the intelligent, living body, as a means of protecting itself, is constantly sending messages, in the form of minor discomfort, to alert you to the fact that if something isn't done, the discomfort will turn into something far more serious; namely, inflammation.

The body doesn't just go straight to the inflammation state when toxins start to accumulate in the tissues. First there are many warning symptoms designed to get your attention and nudge you into action. These symptoms fall under the category of irritation versus the much more painful inflammation. The symptoms of irritation are not serious or even overly painful, but they are bothersome, which is your body's way of getting your attention. Only if these symptoms are ignored and nothing is done to remove the cause of irritation do they develop into something more serious. There are many of these symptoms of irritation and they can go on for years before the inflammation state takes hold. If you are presently dealing with inflammation I am certain that many of these symptoms will be familiar to you because they are the precursor to inflammation.

As one example, a common warning of irritation due to a buildup of toxins is itchiness. The skin is not only the largest organ of the body but it is also an organ of elimination along with the bowels, bladder, and lungs. The body freely and regularly uses the skin's millions of pores to remove toxins from the body, from the top of your head to the bottom of your feet and everything in between. If any area of your skin becomes itchy, that is a classic sign that toxins are being removed and when they reach the surface of the skin, that area becomes irritated. Other symptoms of irritation are lethargy and loss of appetite. Some people will feel queasy or nauseated for no apparent reason and at different times of day. Another is a persistent tickling sensation in the nose. Yet another is to feel jumpy or uneasy or on edge so that you fly off the handle for no apparent reason. If you find yourself uncharacteristically short-tempered or easily aggravated, those are signs of irritation.

Other warning signs of irritation include nervousness, depression, anxiety, and worry, especially when those conditions are out of character for you. You may start to experience headaches or have minor aches and pains in other areas of your body. Difficulty falling asleep or fitful sleep are other indications of irritation. Other classic indicators are coated tongue, bad breath, increased body odor, and sallow complexion, especially dark circles under the eyes. Now you may be thinking right now, "Hey, is anything not a warning signal?" And that's just about right. As I said they are not designed to put you into a state of unbearable pain, but rather are specifically designed to move you to do the right thing so that the state of inflammation does not have to occur.

This is an extremely crucial point in time. What you do at this critical juncture when the body is in a state of irritation will determine whether the irritation and accompanying discomfort merely fades away or accelerates into full blown inflammation and debilitating pain. If the proper corrective steps are taken, to take the burden off of the lymph system, thereby freeing it to cleanse the offending toxins from the body, the symptoms of irritation would simply disappear because their purpose would have been fulfilled—that of alerting you to the situation. And if people had been properly educated as to how to do that—that would be the end of it. Unfortunately that education has been lacking so the automatic, knee-jerk reaction to the symptoms of irritation is to try and suppress them. It's off to the pharmacy for some over-the-counter drugs. Once this action is taken the outcome is predictable and inevitable. The store-bought drugs might lessen the symptoms of discomfort somewhat but without altering the very habits that brought the problem on in the first place, it is only a matter of time before the situation deteriorates into inflammation and the real pain hits and the big guns—the pharmaceuticals—are brought out. It's all downhill from there. The original problem just continues to worsen; more pain means more drugs and stronger drugs. It's a dead end street.

Earlier I promised to supply you with a more reasonable, logical, and plausible explanation for the presence of inflammation and antibodies in the connective tissue than the one associated with the autoimmune theory. We're being asked to believe the preposterous assertion that some nebulous, non-descript, and undetectable "something" draws antibodies to an area of distress in the body. Then once they arrive, finding nothing there to justify their presence, for some unknown reason, and against all rationale, the antibodies start attacking the body's own healthy tissue causing the destructive and painful inflammation associated with disease. If only you knew how impossibly improbable and how laden with indefensible inconsistencies such an outlandish scenario actually is. It flies in the face of everything that affirms the unparalleled intelligence of the dynamic living body.

The very people, who declare that they don't know the cause of Fibromyalgia, Lupus, Arthritis, and Chronic Fatigue Syndrome, and have come up with this illogical **"possible"** fable, are the same ones who have historically and notoriously shunned the study of diet and nutrition. This blunder has left them unaware of the long term repercussions of a poor diet, namely the effects of not effectively and efficiently cleansing the body of wastes (toxins). Unaware of the effect these uneliminated toxins have on healthy tissue they are left in the untenable position of having to defend and cling to this ludicrous and totally speculative autoimmune theory, which they do with stubborn obstinacy.

For some reason these same people are convinced that the solution to Fibromyalgia, Lupus, Arthritis, and Chronic Fatigue Syndrome cannot possibly be simple and straightforward but rather must be deeply complicated, complex, and difficult to figure out. Let me tell you here and now that uneliminated toxins will settle in the tissues causing them to become inflamed. When this happens the incomparable intelligence of the living body, in an all-out effort to protect itself, martials its forces and directs powerful antibodies (white blood cells) to the inflamed area to deal with the situation. The antibodies don't **cause** the inflammation; they are an integral part of the process to **remove** the cause of the inflammation. Doesn't this make infinitely more sense than the convoluted, hypothetical explanation based solely on unprovable conjecture that is the autoimmune theory?

If you were to see a big pile of garbage with flies buzzing all around and feeding on it what would you think if I said, "Will you look at all that garbage those flies dragged in here?" What if I tried to convince you that the flies were responsible for producing the garbage and before they showed up there was no garbage? You would think I was either joking or soon to be chased down by some guys in white with big butterfly nets. It is equally as foolish to suggest that antibodies create inflammation in healthy tissue when in actuality the antibodies are there to reduce and remove the inflammation; which is exactly what they will do if the proper steps are taken to facilitate the process. You are going to learn those proper steps in Part Two of this book.

Inflammation and pain are the means by which the body both attempts to protect itself and alert us to the situation. Sadly, and inaccurately, the medical community regards inflammation as a "disease" entity to be suppressed, but in reality it is a healing process initiated by the body in an effort to reestablish health. Toxins will collect and concentrate in body parts and organs throughout the body, including the connective tissue. When they have accumulated to such an extent as to interfere with normal function or to endanger health, the inflammatory process is utilized to accelerate healing. Any attempt to suppress, interfere with, or interrupt this process only compounds the problem. It has to be treated intelligently, not with toxic, poisonous drugs that interfere with the body's healing effort.

In the beginning of the book I mentioned that there is disagreement about whether or not Fibromyalgia is or is not an inflammatory disease as are Lupus, Arthritis, and Chronic Fatigue Syndrome. Frankly I am perplexed that the medical point of view is that it is not. Of course I shouldn't be surprised, after all, practically everything else associated with Fibromyalgia, Lupus, Arthritis, Chronic Fatigue Syndrome, what they are, how they develop, and how they should be treated from the medical point of view is incorrect so why shouldn't this be as well.

Think of the everywhere-present connective tissue permeating the entirety of the inside of the body, all throughout the muscles, tendons, ligaments, the joints, the organs, holding and supporting everything in place—everything everywhere. When this connective tissue becomes inflamed, depending upon where in the body the inflammation occurs, a different name is given to describe the area of pain and distress. If it's in the tendons, ligaments, organs, or area supporting the organs it's called Lupus. If it is in the joints it's called Arthritis. And if it's in the muscles it's called Fibro-myalgia. It makes no sense and is completely illogical to rule out inflammation when it occurs in the connective tissue just because it's inside the muscles. Plus, if it's not an inflammatory disease, why are anti-inflammatory drugs prescribed?

The overwhelming malaise suffered by those with Chronic Fatigue Syndrome is due to the nonstop expenditure of energy that the body puts forth in the ongoing effort to deal with inflammation and remove the wastes that cause inflammation. It's not only

Fibromyalgia, Lupus, and Arthritis that results in Chronic Fatigue Syndrome; **any** ailment of the body can contribute to it as the body only has a certain amount of energy to go around. More on this shortly.

Three of the symptoms common to Fibromyalgia, Lupus, Arthritis, and Chronic Fatigue Syndrome are pain, malaise, and swollen glands, and all three are part of the intelligent body's attempt to not only protect itself but also to bring to your attention the need for you to take action to support the body's cleansing effort. If at this point you do the right thing, the pain and discomfort will go away, because their **purpose would have been served**. Tragically, because people have not been properly educated to understand what the right thing is, they wind up doing the wrong thing, which all too often means taking drugs to fight the symptoms.

You must understand that drugs do not fix or heal **anything**. Their sole purpose is to fight symptoms, not to overcome the **cause** of the symptoms. Drugs have a threefold negative effect. First, they give you a false sense of security. When the symptoms are masked it tends to give the false impression that the problem itself is being reduced. It isn't. Remember, symptoms are part of the body's warning system, and drugs silence the warnings, so you think nothing is wrong. Second, drugs are themselves, one and all, toxic, so the level of toxins in your body is

increased, which is the last thing you want. Third, drugs actually suppress the activities of the lymph system while giving it even **more** work to do, and that's a bad combination.

We would be well advised to not lose sight of the fact that the pharmaceutical industry, notwithstanding its constant and disingenuous proclamations that it is tirelessly seeking "cures," is doing nothing of the kind. One of the biggest mistakes you will ever make this lifetime is to think that the pharmaceutical industry cares anything whatsoever about you other than how it might extract more money out of your purse or wallet. I know how heartless, cold, and cynical this is to say but pain is the pharmaceutical industry's stock in trade; it no more wants to find the "cure" for pain than America wants to elevate Osama Bin Laden to sainthood status. Your misery translates into profits. The pharmaceutical industry has the greatest net profits of any industry in the United States[34] and that is directly attributed to the fact that so many millions of people are in pain. The industry **needs** pain for its very survival and is perfectly content to keep pumping out new drugs to fight symptoms and raking in the money.

When I say that the pharmaceutical industry busies itself with pumping out new drugs, that is an understatement. At present, there are 3.4 **billion** prescriptions written and dispensed in the United States every year,[34A] which translates into 12 prescriptions each for every man, woman, and child in the country! This is an all-time high and is nearly **double** the number of prescriptions purchased only a decade ago. These billions of prescriptions generate astronomical amounts of money because they are very expensive.

One of the key reasons drug prices in the United States are **the most** expensive in the world is because every developed country, except the United States, regulates the prices that drug makers can charge consumers. The U.S. government has chosen not to do this, mainly because of effective drug-industry lobbying. That is one reason why the industry can get away with charging such obscene prices, such as **over $1,000 a month** for Humira, a drug for Rheumatoid Arthritis.[34B] And that's not the only one; there are plenty of drugs that cost over $1,000 a month.

The interminably long list of drugs for pain constantly changes as some are dropped for either causing harm or death only to be replaced with the latest one to come off the assembly line. In September, 2004, the "blockbuster pain reliever" Vioxx, for Arthritis pain, was taken off the market after it was blamed for over 27,000 heart attacks and sudden cardiac deaths.[35] This was nothing more than a temporary inconvenience for the pharmaceutical industry which simply focuses on other drugs or on new drugs until such time that **they** fall by the wayside once their deadliness is determined. Sure it's a shame about the 27,000 victims but it had a nice five year run and made several billion dollars before the bodies started piling up.

Like it or not, regardless of the human toll, for the pharmaceutical industry, it's all about the money, not your health. *The Wall Street Journal* reported that "Internal e-mails and other documents from Merck & Co. (the makers of Vioxx) show the company fought for years to keep safety concerns from undermining the drug's commercial prospects."[35A] Kind of warms your heart doesn't it?

The Vioxx scandal brought to light in a very unsettling way just how perilously unstable the entire system of drugging is in relying so heavily on them to combat pain. Vioxx belongs to a class of drugs called COX-2 inhibitors, hailed when they were first introduced, as a "miracle breakthrough in pain relief" because they did not harm the lining of the stomach or cause ulcers the way aspirin and other traditional treatments could. As Vioxx, along with Bextra and Celebrex (other COX-2 miracles), fell by the wayside due to their deadliness, tens of millions of people were left in a lurch as they went to their doctors in a panic only to be told that they were as confused and caught by surprise as everyone else.

Many physicians relied very heavily on the COX-2s as their standard treatment for arthritis pain. As the reputation for these drugs started to crumble like a sand castle being hit by waves, some patients were recommended to take other anti-inflammatory drugs for their arthritis pain. Two such drugs were Remicade and Methotrexate, and it is with these two drugs that I can most clearly and dramatically illustrate to you the insanity associated with the mechanical reliance on drugs as the automatic treatment of choice in dealing with pain.

As the Vioxx/Bextra/Celebrex debacle played itself out, Remicade and Methotrexate also found themselves in the news as well. In August, 2004 it was reported that there were 25 patient deaths and 26 cases of serious harm linked to the use of Methotrexate in the UK.[35B] In October, 2004 it was reported that patients taking Remicade suffered a type of cancer, lymphoma, at three times the rate of the general public.[35C] Now hold on to your seat friend, because this stuff just can't be made up. In November, 2004 I read this headline: **"Arthritis Improves with Remicade plus Methotrexate."**[35D]

Never mind the rhetoric from the "experts," what does your common sense tell you about the declaration that Remicade can give you cancer, Methotrexate can **kill** you, but when taken together they will help you? Such an assertion is too strange even for fiction. Mark Twain once said, "Why shouldn't truth be stranger than fiction? Fiction, after all, has to make sense."

The *Washington Post* reported on a study that appeared in the *Journal of the American Medical*

Association revealing that two million people are seriously injured every year as a result of taking prescription drugs.[35E] These injuries are not because of accidents, but rather as a result of the toxic nature of the drugs taken properly and according to the directions that accompany the prescriptions.

One of the greatest tragedies this country has ever had to bear was the World Trade Center catastrophe. Nearly 3,000 people tragically perished. I doubt if there is a single person in the entire United States not aware of those deaths. I wonder how many people are equally aware, that according to the study referred to above, 106,000 people die every year from taking prescription drugs **correctly**. Again, I'm not talking about accidents, which would, according to the study, cause the number to **double**; I'm talking about deaths exclusively as a result of taking the correct drugs in the correct manner in which they were designed to be taken. We are talking about more deaths than breast cancer, prostate cancer, and AIDS combined! That is **35 times** the number of deaths at the World Trade Center and it happens **every year**! Where's the outrage for that?

Now, just because I am taking such a strong stand in opposition to drugs I don't want to imply that I am some inflexible fanatic that thinks all drugs should be avoided at all times. I know full well that emergency situations require emergency measures and when someone is in unrelenting pain drugs bring temporary relief.

I am endeavoring to present the larger picture here of **why** a person is in pain in the first place and what can be done to address and alleviate the cause, removing the necessity for drugs. At present all emphasis and research is on finding "new and better" drugs to help people cope, and nothing is being done to mitigate the problem itself. When the one and only option is drugs it essentially condemns people with Fibromyalgia, Lupus, Arthritis, and Chronic Fatigue Syndrome to a lifetime of drug taking.

The truly sad part is that not only do the drugs not help remove the problem, but they actually make it worse. Guess what the COX-2s were designed and intended to do? **Suppress** the immune system. To suppress it. When was the last time you heard advice, from **anyone**, to **weaken** your immune system in order to get well? How much more evidence do you need to illustrate that these folks simply don't know what they're doing and are fumbling around in the dark? The absolute number one, most urgent need for life to continue is air; six minutes without it means death. Can you imagine a circumstance where it would be best to **decrease** your ability to inhale and exhale? No! That's not logical. Not only would it be illogical, even foolhardy, to recommend someone diminish the effectivelness of their immune system's activities, it would be downright idiotic to suggest doing so at the time of greatest need when the person is sick or in pain and in need of the immune system working unrestrict-ed and at its highest possible capacity. But that is pre-cisely what is done on a routine basis in this country when people are in pain; they are given drugs to specifically hinder the activities of the immune sys-tem. Is it any wonder that pain remains the number one health complaint in the United States and the statistics associated with pain increase **every** year?

There is a better way; a less harmful, less expen-sive, more sensible, more natural way to deal with pain that you will never, ever hear about from the avaricious pharmaceutical industry. It is a strategy that revolves around a greater understanding, admiration, and reverence for the remarkable living body and its unequaled healing abilities. It is a strategy that revolves around strengthening and supporting the lymph system so it can unleash its healing power, not poisoning it with dangerous, toxic drugs that thwart its efforts. Doesn't it make much more sense to take steps that will reduce pain so that less and less drugs are necessary until they can be discontinued altogether? Even if it takes a year or more to completely be free of the drugs, isn't that better than knowing that drugs will have to be taken daily for the rest of your life?

Fibromyalgia, Lupus, Arthritis, and Chronic Fatigue Syndrome don't just sneak up on you. It's not as though you go to bed one night with no symptoms and wake up in the morning with a full-blown case. No, it's a slow, drawn-out process that progressively worsens over time if proper measures aren't taken. I want you to think about your own experience. Whether it was one year ago or 10 years ago, think about the very first time you were aware that something wasn't quite right. Maybe you started to have some minor aches and pains that would come and go for no obvious reason. Perhaps you started to notice with increasing regularity that you felt tired around midmorning or midafternoon. Maybe you started to feel "cranky" or irritated for no apparent reason, which was completely out of character for you. Maybe you just generally felt out of sorts, unable to put your finger on exactly what was going on. All symptoms of irritation.

Can you recall what you did or thought about those symptoms at the time? Were they minor enough that you just shrugged them off? Did you take note of the symptoms but not give them too much attention? Did you attribute them to time and age, thinking, as many people do, that at some point something has to start to hurt? Did you go to the doctor for a checkup? Or did you figure that since the symptoms weren't chronic they would take care of themselves?

What about as time went by and you noticed that the symptoms which were minor and infrequent at first were becoming more intense, occurring more frequently and lasting longer? What did you do then? Did you make any lifestyle changes? Did you change your diet or exercise more or work less or seek help in any way? Did you decide to "take something" from over the counter to increase your pep or reduce your pain? Did you obtain some kind of prescription drug?

Whatever you did then, I wonder if you would have done anything differently had you known about your lymph system and the steps you could have taken to cleanse and strengthen it. Because I can tell you that if you did do then what you are going to have the opportunity to do now with the information in this book, well....you wouldn't be in need of this book, because the problem would not have persisted. The body's warnings would have been heeded, the proper steps would have been taken, and the symptoms would have gone away.

Perhaps you're a bit skeptical about what I'm saying as I describe with such certainty what you can achieve by optimizing the activities of your lymph system. Especially if you have been long in your suffering. All I can ask is that you try what I am suggesting and see for yourself. After all, what if I'm right? What if you really can get on top of this thing and live a more pain-free life by utilizing the steps that I'm going to suggest? Wouldn't it be worth it? And when you see the simplicity of what I am proposing you do, I think you'll see that it is indeed worth the effort even if you enjoy only a moderate improvement at first.

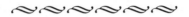

In addition to the people I have seen overcome Fibromyalgia, Lupus, Arthritis, and Chronic Fatigue Syndrome by the cleansing and strengthening of their lymph system, there is one particularly convincing piece of evidence that is the basis for my confidence and assuredness. It stands as an impressive testimony to the power of the lymph system and what it can achieve given the opportunity.

Do you recall when I mentioned earlier that I had firsthand knowledge of the frustration associated with having a serious problem with the body and being told by the experts that they had no idea what was wrong? In 1986 the first **FIT FOR LIFE** book had been published, and it literally broke all records as it skyrocketed to the top of all the bestseller lists. I was on top of the world. Not only was I enjoying supremely good health, due to living the very principles the book outlined, but millions of other people were enjoying a newfound health as well, thanks to the book. I had the satisfaction of knowing that I was helping others as I helped myself, fulfilling the ancient creed to "Love your neighbor as yourself." I was enjoying success on all levels—personally, professionally, and financially.

Then, at the height of my prosperity, for no apparent reason, the muscles in my arms and legs started to wither. It was frightening beyond any description I could give. It started slowly at first with a slight limp in my right leg and an almost imperceptible weakness in my hands. But month after month it became worse and worse, with no letup in sight. The limp became more pronounced, and I started to have difficulty grasping and lifting even lightweight objects with my arms and hands. I was, to put it mildly, **freaking out**.

I spent the next **three and a half years** traveling all over the United States, going to numerous experts in a wide range of disciplines in a desperate attempt to find out what the heck was going on. Nothing. **Nothing**! No one could give me even the slightest hint about what was causing my muscles to atrophy. I was poked, prodded, and tested. I gave blood, had CAT scans, and MRIs. You name it, I tried it. I even had all the mercury removed from my teeth because it was suggested that that might be the culprit. Everywhere I went, all over the country for three and a half years as my condition became progressively worse, the only thing I heard was, "All our tests show you to be in particularly good health. Well, except for this muscle thing."

The English language does not provide words to sufficiently relate to you what it felt like to wake up every morning wondering how much worse my condition would be that day. And not having even a clue about what was causing the deterioration was unbearable.

Then in 1989 I talked to someone who was going through the **exact same thing himself**. The only difference was that he had been dealing with it for a longer time, and it had progressed to the point where he was confined to a wheelchair. After I told him what my symptoms were, which coincided with his own at the beginning of his deterioration, he asked me when my muscles first started to deteriorate. After I told him it had started in 1986, he said without the slightest hesitation, "Well, then you must have been somewhere in Vietnam in 1966." Since I had been stationed in Vietnam for the entire year of 1966 while serving in the Air Force, I asked him how on Earth he could possibly have known that.

To this day, over 15 years later, his answer still sends chills up my spine and adrenaline through my veins. Following is the substance of what he told me as I sat in stunned silence with my mind reeling as the blinding realization of the cause of my predicament became apparent. I had a condition known as peripheral neuropathy, brought on by exposure to Agent Orange while I was in Vietnam. A derivative of Agent Orange is dioxin, which is considered to be the most toxic human-made poison ever formulated. Agent Orange was thought to be safe when 11 million gallons of it was dumped onto the jungles of Vietnam in the hope of wiping out all foliage so the Viet Cong would have nowhere to hide. It didn't work, but it did poison thousands of people. And I was one of them.

It was thought to be safe at the time because it hadn't been tested for long enough. You see, Agent Orange sits in the body for **20 years** incubating and percolating before you even have an idea of the harm that it causes. After 20 years, among the long list of dreadful problems it causes, peripheral neuropathy starts to become apparent. First the hands, arms, and legs start to deteriorate, then it affects the muscles of the torso, and five years after deterioration starts (which, remember, is 20 years after exposure) those with peripheral neuropathy are either immobilized in a wheelchair or dead.

This man knew so much about the subject because he was the president of the Agent Orange Support Group in the United States. He told me that my story was identical to hundreds of others. Twenty years after exposure, deterioration started, and five years later they were in a wheelchair (as he was) or dead.

If I live to be a thousand years old I will never be able to erase from my mind what he told me next. It has been burned into my memory as though with a branding iron. After repeating that no one had made it past five years from the time deterioration started, he said almost casually, considering what he was saying, that "I probably had about 18 months left." At first I

was so filled with a combination of fear, rage, and disbelief that I couldn't move or speak, because I was
paralyzed by his statement. Actually, I almost passed
out. But deep inside of me something was indignantly
screaming out, "**What?! WHAT?! You have to be
kidding me!**" So, in other words, after spending nearly 20 years dedicated to studying health I was to die or
be completely paralyzed in a year and a half from
being poisoned nearly a quarter of a century earlier?

Over that next year and a half I went through various stages of mental states, everything from the cry of
the victim—"Why me?"—to the loftier, "I guess this
is what God wants for me." But the dreaded five-year
deadline came and went, and I was still standing. In
fact, as I am writing this it has been **19 years** since
deterioration started, and I am one of, if not **the**
longest known survivor of Agent Orange-induced
peripheral neuropathy to still be walking around on his
own without assistance. True, I continue to have obvious lingering damage in that I walk with a significant
limp, and I must struggle with both arms and hands
just to lift a glass of water to my mouth, or to perform
any number of simple activities that even a small child
could perform with only one hand, but I'm alive! And
other than the damage to my muscles I am in excellent
health.

You've probably heard people who are dealing
with seemingly unbearable challenges say something

to the effect of, "Everything happens for a reason." As the years went by and my condition slowly but inexorably progressed, I very much wanted to know the higher reason and meaning for what I was going through. There had to be a higher, deeper purpose. Why would someone who was able to learn and share principles of health that helped millions of people all over the world live longer, healthier lives be saddled with such a devastating affliction of the body?

Gradually, the answer became crystal clear to me. Of the hundreds of people who have died or have been confined to a wheelchair, what was it about me that was the determining factor in my being spared? Luck? No way. It was my lymph system. You see, I was exposed to Agent Orange in 1966, and my muscles didn't start to wither until 1986, but in 1970 (only four years after exposure) I started to conscientiously care for my lymph system. Not because of the Agent Orange; I wouldn't even know I was exposed for another 16 years. No, I started to clean my lymph system to help me with the pain and other health problems I was trying to overcome. Little did I know at the time that that effort would wind up saving my life! My body had a 16-year head start on battling the effects of the poisoning that others with peripheral neuropathy did not have, and that made the difference.

I have taken on as my personal mission the goal of bringing to people's awareness the seemingly miraculous health benefits that can be realized as a result of the proper care and treatment of their lymph system. For most people it's a brand-new subject, one with which they are not at all familiar. Because an understanding of the lymph system is so far removed from their mind, people want to have some kind of dramatic proof or substantiation of its worthiness. Especially considering that someone is always coming up with the latest, greatest breakthrough that promises to put everything else to shame as it transforms lives. They're not interested in speculation. They want to hear about what is **known**. They don't want guesswork. They want evidence based on life experiences.

I can speak with such conviction and certainty about what can be expected for those who properly care for their lymph systems because in my case, doing so saved my life. What's more powerful than that? Can you see that if my lymph system was successful in overcoming the effects of the most deadly toxin in existence, then your lymph system will surely have an easier time of it in dealing with the normal, everyday toxins produced in your body that are the cause of your Fibromyalgia, Lupus, Arthritis, or Chronic Fatigue Syndrome? All you have to do is take the steps to unleash your body's own remarkable cleansing and healing capabilities.

It saddens me when I hear people say things like "My body is my enemy" or "My body is conspiring against me." Nothing in the entire world could be further from the truth. Your body is your greatest ally. It's just a matter of learning how to get out of its way so it can do what it is already trying to do. We should be in a constant state of astonishment about the intelligence of our body, yet we take it largely for granted. We must begin to nurture a newfound appreciation and respect for the unparalleled ability to heal that our body possesses.

If you would indulge me, I would like to end this part of the book with one last water-related analogy. Picture a man out on the water, far from land, in a rowboat. He has no oars, no paddles, nothing to move the boat through the water to the land. The sides of the boat are too high for him to paddle with his hands, so he is stuck out there on the water, and so he perishes. He dies for want of some means to carry him to land. How ironic and senseless would his death be if all the while a perfectly good motor was on the back of the boat that he never noticed and therefore never used? He could have, at any time, fired up the motor and taken himself to shore and safety instead of dying needlessly.

Your lymph system is that motor, and you can fire it up anytime you want to and rescue yourself from the effects of Fibromyalgia, Lupus, Arthritis, and Chronic Fatigue Syndrome. It is waiting patiently for you to give it the opportunity to do what it has been specifically designed to do. Of course the question of the moment is, "How exactly do I go about firing up my lymph system and thereby coming to my own rescue?" That, dear friend, is the subject of the remainder of the book.

PART TWO

THE SOLUTION

THE SOLUTION

INTRODUCTION TO

THE THREE STEPS TO RECOVERY

We are here to eat. That's right, we humans are eating machines. Most of the internal organs of our body are involved in one way or another in the three primary activities of life. Remember? Taking in food, metabolism, and elimination of waste. Food plays a central role in everyone's life. We eat approximately every four hours (while awake) and in many cases even more frequently. To most people, going for a full day without eating a single bite of food is about as appealing as falling down a flight of stairs.

Eating isn't something that is optional. We **must** eat, or we'll die. Period. That's not open for debate.

Food, along with water and air, are the three indispensable requirements for life to continue. It is from the food we eat that we obtain not only the nutrients that the body needs to build, repair, and maintain tissue but also the energy necessary to conduct the countless number of activities that the body performs every moment. And so in a lifetime we each eat approximately 70 tons of food. That seems implausible, does it not, that our body, which on average weighs somewhere between 100 and 200 pounds, will consume in the neighborhood of 140,000 pounds?

Try to envision the time, effort, and energy required over a lifetime merely to gather, prepare, and consume all of that food. Then once it is chewed up and swallowed the body has to process it, extract what it needs from it, deliver the nutrients and energy to all the cells, and eliminate the waste that is left. Seventy tons' worth! Truly an astounding accomplishment.

It is quite impossible to discuss the subject of food and not also include the subject of energy in that discussion. Energy is the one essential, can't-do-without ingredient that fuels absolutely every last activity of the living body, large or small. When energy is in abundance, life is so much more enjoyable. When energy is in short supply, life becomes tedious. When energy is gone entirely, life is over. One thing I have never, ever heard is people complaining about having too much energy. You just don't hear comments like,

"Doggone it, I'm sick and tired of having to figure out what to do with all this energy."

Energy truly is the essence of life. It is our most precious commodity. That's because we could do **nothing** without it. It's important to understand that since energy is required for literally every action of the living body, every measure available to us must be taken to conserve it when possible and not waste any needlessly. When we awaken in the morning we have our full complement of energy for that day, which was built up while we slept. It takes energy to blink your eyes, to stand up or sit down, to pick up a pencil. Obviously it takes way more energy to run a marathon than it does to brush your teeth, but the body's energy reserves are being steadily used up either in large allotments or small. And when the day's supply is used up, that's it. When that happens before the day's activities are completed, you start to hear people complain: "I am really beat" or "Man, I'm so tired I can't move" or "I can't believe it's only 2:00, I'm wasted" or any number of other comments indicating that a person is out of energy.

Why do you think so many people rely on coffee or cola drinks or other caffeinated products? Some even purchase over-the-counter "pick-me-ups" which artificially stimulate— anything to get through the day. But those things all take their toll. It's not true energy. The "lift" people feel is actually the body's using its resources to speed up and eliminate what it perceives as an irritant or a poison in the system. Then there's the inevitable drop, which requires more, even stronger stimulants. It is a cycle that is hard to break and that takes its toll on the body in the long run.

You can compare the use of a day's energy to the spending of money. If you have a thousand dollars to last you for a set period of time, you can either spend it in big chunks or small. If you run out before the time comes when you get more money, you may have to borrow some to see you through. But it's not free. You have to pay the borrowed money back, usually with interest. If you keep doing that, you never catch up and wind up in permanent debt. The same thing can happen in terms of your energy. The difference is that the debt of energy translates into a lower state of health.

So want to take a wild guess about what activity of the body uses more energy than any other? It in fact uses more energy than all other uses **combined**. Give up? Digestion! Think about this: Everything you do during your entire life, and I mean everything, all of which requires energy, all added together will not use the amount of energy that will be used to digest and metabolize the 70 tons of food you will eat. Food in the stomach is a number-one priority for the body. Food just can't sit around in the stomach. The body immediately allocates whatever energy is necessary to initiate the digestive process that starts in the stomach.

Do you ever feel tired after a meal? Of course you do. Everyone does. And the bigger the meal, the more tired you are. What did you do right after eating dinner last Thanksgiving, look for your running shoes or a couch? Is there anyone who does not know what the "afternoon siesta" is? People eat a big lunch and then have to take a nap.

The key to success in overcoming the pain of Fibromyalgia, Lupus, Arthritis, and Chronic Fatigue Syndrome, and other forms of pain, hinges on the amount of energy that is regularly freed from the digestive tract and made available for use by the lymph system to extract toxins from the connective tissue and remove them from the body.

To repeat:

The key to success in overcoming the pain of Fibromyalgia, Lupus, Arthritis, and Chronic Fatigue Syndrome, and other forms of pain, hinges on the amount of energy that is regularly freed from the digestive tract and made available for use by the lymph system to extract toxins from the connective tissue and remove them from the body.

Do you recall the earlier point that every malady suffered by the human body can ultimately be traced back to how effectively and efficiently food is digested in the stomach? Whether it's Fibromyalgia, Lupus, Arthritis, Chronic Fatigue Syndrome, heart disease, cancer, diabetes, headaches—you name it—everything starts with how well food is digested and how quickly it leaves the stomach. That's the starting point. Obviously if food is in the stomach for three hours rather than seven or eight hours, a whole lot less energy is going to be required to deal with it and move it on its way through to the intestines.

The plain truth is that more energy is unnecessarily squandered in the stomach than by any other cause. There is a way of eating that streamlines digestion, thereby freeing energy, and there is a way that hinders and prolongs digestion, thereby squandering energy. The simple equation is this: The less energy that is used in the number-one priority of digestion, the more will be available for the extraction and removal of toxins from the body. It must be strange indeed if all of this is new to you to learn that your recovery from Fibromyalgia, Lupus, Arthritis, and Chronic Fatigue Syndrome begins in your stomach. But strange though it may be, that's the case.

The difference between success and failure lies in your willingness to make some simple yet strategic dietary changes that result in the freeing of energy from the energy-intensive digestive process. That "found" energy is automatically redirected by the intelligent body to the lymph system so it can fuel the all-important process of flushing toxins from the body.

My contention is that the manner in which you have eaten your entire life, in some cases from infancy, is the cause of your present predicament, so a change in those dietary habits which brought on the problem in the first place must be undertaken.

Before going even one word further I want to allay any concerns you may be harboring that you are going to be eating a diet of wood chips and grass clippings washed down with mineral water. You can put that right out of your mind. Eating plays far too big a role in our life for it to become a clinical endeavor of calorie counting, portion measuring, and deprivation.

The eating experience **must** remain a joyous one, or else the entire process of recovery becomes a forced march of punishment rather than an enjoyable and pleasurable experience. Besides, being a confirmed, dyed-in-the-wool foodaholic who loves food and loves to eat, I would never be associated with an eating plan based on restriction and deprivation that constantly leaves you hungry, bored, and wanting more. No food groups are excluded, no off-the-wall practices that fly in the face of reason, no long, complicated list of do's, don'ts, can'ts and nevers. Changes will be required, yes, but I think you'll be not only surprised but also encouraged by an eating plan that is simple, straightforward, sensible, and satisfying.

It has been my experience over the years that most

people do not take into account that the human digestive system has some very definite limitations. The digestive system **is** extraordinary in what it accomplishes and will always make the greatest effort possible under all circumstances, even when forced to deal with more than what it is designed to handle. But constantly being pushed beyond its limitations inevitably leads to problems. Most people are laboring under the false impression that they can eat any kind of food at any time day or night in any combination and the body will just handle it. That is a primary reason why we lead the world in the degenerative diseases and why so many people suffer with Fibromyalgia, Lupus, Arthritis, and Chronic Fatigue Syndrome.

You wouldn't push your muscular/skeletal system beyond its limits by asking it to pick up and move cars for a living would you? Of course not. You know that the muscles are able to lift only a certain amount of weight and no more. But the digestive system is asked daily, in a manner of speaking, to lift more than it can carry. I don't know where on Earth people got the idea that they could eat absolutely any food they desire at any time and as long as it's chewed up and swallowed, it will be digested and turned into healthy cell structure. It won't!

Why do you think billions and billions of dollars are spent every year on digestive aids? Over-the-counter and prescription drugs for stomachaches, indigestion, gas, bloating, flatulence, acid stomach, heartburn, acid reflux, and ulcers account for some of the pharmaceutical industry's greatest income. Why are so many drugs necessary for doing something as normal and natural as eating?

As an aside, I'm going to indulge myself and take this opportunity to mention one of my all-time favorite pet peeves: the stomach virus, one of the most preposterous and moronic bits of idiocy ever to be foisted onto an unsuspecting public. As if there actually was some microscopic organism that existed for the sole purpose of finding its way into the stomachs of human beings for the singular purpose of making its host nauseous. Right; and cigarettes don't contribute to lung cancer and Charlton Heston doesn't own a gun. Oh, yeah, and politicians never lie. The term *stomach virus* has become a part of everyday vocabulary, especially in sports.

Typically, there will be some 350-pound football player on the sideline barfing his guts out, and the announcer will say, "Looks like ol' Bubba has himself a stomach virus." No mention of Bubba's plundering assault at the food trough before the game. Have you ever seen what some of these guys eat right before hitting the field? Sometimes a player will eat enough food to feed a small country. Then when some 280-pound tackle lays a hit on him that feels as if a tree fell on top of him, he starts throwing up and the announcer says he has a stomach virus. When someone throws up a side of beef, six buckets of fried chicken, and a wheelbarrow full of French fries, it's not because of some microscopic scrap of protoplasm one billionth the size of a single cell. It's because of some dietary indiscretion.

I'd be willing to bet that the entire stomach virus business was started by medical doctors who made it a point never to study nutrition. Confronted with the task of explaining something as simple and obvious as stomach upsets and vomiting, dumbfounded and bewildered graduates of one of the medical colleges not interested in teaching nutrition simply fall back on their favorite scapegoat: "Oh, it must be a stomach virus."

Digestive problems are one of the pharmaceutical industry's biggest moneymakers every year. You don't think that's a coincidence, do you? The reason, as outrageously absurd as it may sound, is because people have never been taught how to eat. Now obviously I don't mean they have never learned how to get food into their mouth. I think we can all agree that has been learned perfectly well. What I mean is that people have never learned how to eat in such a way that not only satisfies the **desire** to eat and eat well but also honors and supports the digestive system's limitations.

Many years ago, in the early 1970s, I remember

reading an article, the title of which threw me at first because at the time I couldn't relate to it. It was entitled, "Food, the One True Medicine for Man." (I guess the authors didn't know there were women back then). I was taken aback because I associated food with something yummy and pleasurable and medicine with being sick. Medicine was some yucky-tasting concoction I would have to swallow while I held my nose. Food was definitely not medicine. Of course reading the article gave me a different perspective.

I can't remember exactly what the article said, but I remember its essential content. In fact I could easily see myself writing such an article. The basic message was that the type and quality of the food we eat and the manner in which we eat it can make us sick. And by altering the type and quality of the food we eat and the manner in which we eat it, it can make us well again. The Three Steps to Recovery that follow this introduction are specifically designed to support and assist your body in its ongoing effort to recapture health.

The key to success revolves around some specific dietary maneuvering. So it's not as though the foods you are presently eating are replaced by other foods or that you have to become a vegetarian or that you can't eat when you are hungry or that you must dramatically alter your lifestyle. Instead, there are definite ways to manipulate what you eat, when you eat, and how you eat, in such a way as to minimize the amount of time food is in your stomach gobbling up the precious energy that will instead be used to maximize the efforts of your lymph system.

Basically I am talking about some fine-tuning. It's like tuning in some music on a radio station. If you want to listen to 102.5 and the radio is tuned to 102.4 or 102.6, there will be scratching interference, and the music will not sound very good. But as soon as you move the dial ever so slightly to 102.5, everything clears up, and the music comes in loud and clear. That's all you're going to be doing with your diet— some fine-tuning. You'll be amazed at what a big difference a little adjustment makes.

In 1923 there were 12 food groups. In 1941 it was lowered to seven food groups, and by 1960 it was condensed to the four food groups that are still in effect today. Even though the four-food-group model is a far sight simpler than the old 12-food-group approach, still, considerable confusion, disagreement, and controversy surrounding the four-food-group approach to eating persists. I'm going to simplify it for you. For the purposes of this book and your effort to overcome Fibromyalgia, Lupus, Arthritis, and Chronic Fatigue Syndrome, you will need to concern yourself with only two food groups.

Let us not forget why we humans need to eat in the first place. Remember? **To stay alive**. Yes, eating food is a tasty and enjoyable part of life. Sitting down with family and friends to a table full of delectable goodies is most definitely a great pleasure that brings people together and promotes camaraderie and friendship. But all the pleasure and friendship and good that comes from eating and sharing food is secondary to staying alive, the primary reason for eating food.

Life is, after all, the most supreme gift of gifts. One of my favorite quotes comes from the renowned philosopher and author William Blake, who said, "Everything that lives is holy, life delights in life." I love that last part. Only four words, but they speak volumes. "Life delights in life." What could be more truthful and profound than that? Life delights in life.

As scientists, astronomers, and astronauts explore the outer reaches of our universe with the most technologically advanced equipment ever produced and assembled, the one element most conspicuously missing from their exploration of space is life. No life can be found anywhere, even trillions of miles out in any direction. In fact, it appears that all the life that exists in the entirety of our universe is concentrated right here on our little planet Earth.

Can you even imagine what it would be like if one of the probes that NASA sends to Mars sent back a picture of a flower growing out of the ground? It would be the most momentous discovery in all the history of life on this planet. That's if one flower was to be found. Look around on this planet and you can't help but see life bursting and teeming at every turn. Even in the most desolate and forbidding parts of planet Earth, where temperatures may climb to over 120 degrees or drop to 100 degrees below freezing, life is still to be found. Parts of our planet have such prodigious concentrations of flora and fauna that thousands and thousands of species of life have yet to be isolated and named. How truly special and unique this planet of life is, and how blessed we are to be a part of its unfolding.

Since, as Mr. Blake so eloquently and elegantly stated, "Life delights in life," I want to ask you a question. Inasmuch as we know that without a doubt we **must** eat food in order to prolong and support the great gift of life, which type of food do you think would be best for the living body—food that is alive or food that is dead? No, it's not a trick question; it's more like what is referred to as a "no-brainer." And you don't have to be a scientist or nutritionist to answer. You merely have to use your common sense. Of course you must be thinking, "What an imbecilic question! Obviously living food would be superior to dead food. Why even ask?"

You may be shocked to learn that the diet consumed by most people is very heavily predominated by food that has had all the life in it destroyed before it is eaten. In fact, and please do not take what I'm about to say personally, because I don't want to come across as harsh or insulting, but in all likelihood **you** are one of those people, and you are in the majority. Having never met you, I can still safely make such a statement because were you not one of those who eat far more food that is no longer living than food that is, you would probably not be reading a book on how to overcome pain.

An extremely simple, easy, and straightforward way exists for you to prove one way or the other if I am correct in my assumption that your diet is most likely predominated by food that is not living. Before telling you how to go about proving that for yourself, I want to be certain that you know exactly what determines whether or not a food is living.

In what certainly has to be one of the most remarkable illustrations of the incomprehensible intelligence that governs our life, we humans actually remove from our environment living matter that we chew up and swallow, and it in turn becomes part of our body. It is at one and the same time implausible, yet unimaginably ingenious. We are, in the truest sense possible, kept alive by the constant eating of foodstuffs taken from the environment. And it has been so designed that the food we eat contains not only the building blocks of our body and the energy source to fuel every activity but also an essential component that actually digests the food when it reaches the stomach. This essential component is the life essence of not only the food but astonishingly of **everything else in existence that exhibits life**. What is this miraculous component? Tiny chemical proteins called *enzymes*.

In all likelihood you have heard of enzymes, but did you know that every living thing on this planet that is bursting with life is alive because of enzymes? Every plant, every animal, and every human being is alive because of enzymes. If not for them the planet Earth would be as lifeless and barren as Mars.

So here are the only two food groups from which you will make all of your food choices. The first group consists of the foods that are alive; in other words, the food's full complement of enzymes is intact, totally ready and capable of performing that ever so important task of digestion in the stomach. The second group consists of those foods which have had their enzymes destroyed, thereby rendering the food dead, which forces the body to manufacture its **own** enzymes in order to digest the food. Enzyme-rich foods require a minimum amount of digestive energy from the body, which is precisely the goal we wish to achieve. Enzyme-depleted foods require a massive amount of digestive energy from the body, which is precisely what we wish to avoid.

Considering that effective and efficient digestion of food in the stomach is crucial to the effort of overcoming Fibromyalgia, Lupus, Arthritis, and Chronic Fatigue Syndrome and preventing their return, it stands to reason that enzyme-rich foods would be the food of choice for anyone wishing to live a pain-free, disease-free life.

So the next logical question would have to be, "How are enzymes destroyed?" Heat! Heat wipes them out. As a matter of fact, at 118 degrees all enzymes are destroyed. I don't mean that they are weakened or degraded; at 118 degrees they are obliterated. Foods that are processed and packaged and/or prepared by cooking have had their enzymes destroyed, because the temperature to process or pasteurize or cook a food is far, far in excess of 118 degrees. This does not mean that the food is not digested, because one way or another **all** food must go through the initial stages of digestion in the stomach. What it does mean is that the food will be forced to stay in the stomach for an inordinate length of time, which, number one, squanders huge amounts of energy and overtaxes the body's resources, and two, gives rise to the numerous digestive disorders mentioned earlier.

Here then is the simple test you can give yourself to see if you are indeed eating less food that is alive than food that isn't. Draw a line down the middle of a piece of paper from top to bottom. Then for a period of one day or three days or a week write down absolutely everything you eat, leaving out nothing even if it was only one bite of something. On the left side list those foods that have had the enzymes destroyed either by processing or cooking, and on the right side list the foods that had the enzymes intact.

Let me help you out on this. On the right side of your sheet the only foods that will be listed are uncooked and unprocessed in any way. That means all fruits, vegetables, nuts, seeds, and juices. And that's it. Now remember, **uncooked**. The fruit must be fresh, not fruit cocktail from a can or otherwise cooked. The vegetables must also be raw, as in a salad. Same with the nuts and seeds—not roasted. And the juices can't be pasteurized. The left side of the sheet will be everything else.

As an example, if for breakfast you have bacon and eggs, toast and coffee, or pancakes and hash browns or oatmeal and a bagel, or a Pop tart and a glass of milk, all of it goes on the left side. Or maybe you conscientiously had a bowl of bran or wheat flake cereal, advertised that they "may" lower cholesterol, with nonfat milk. Yes, they are better than those vile atrocities such as Fruit Loops or Lucky Charms that are so soaked in chemical dyes and additives, processed sugar, and preservatives that rats will eat the box and leave the contents. But the less objectionable flake cereals and the milk are heated at temperatures so intense that nothing living could possibly survive. Certainly not the delicate enzymes and nutrients that are so vital to life. List it all on the left side.

If you should have half a grapefruit and some orange juice or a fruit salad, they will all go on the right side. Remember, the orange juice has to be **unpasteurized** to count as fresh. That leaves out all those cartons of orange juice advertised as "pure and natural Florida sunshine" or some other slogan to persuade you to drink orange juice. They are all heated to temperatures way above 118 degrees, so the enzymes have been burnt away. The advertisers want you to think it's fresh and natural, but they are neither. In the body, pasteurized orange juice is pure all right—pure acid. Same with other fruit juices bought in bottles and cartons. If they're pasteurized, they are devoid of enzymes.

Do the same thing with lunch and dinner. Only what is uncooked and unprocessed goes on the right side of your list. All the bread and butter, pasta, meat, chicken, fish, or dairy products, baked potatoes, milk, soda, and coffee—all go on the left. The salad goes on the right. Got the picture?

By now some people reading this have to be saying something to the effect of, "Hey wait just a gol-dern minute! If you're telling me I have to become a raw fooder and never eat anything cooked, you're nuts. I'd rather take my chances with drugs." Rest assured, I am definitely **not** suggesting that you must eat only uncooked food. I am only trying to make a point. The point being that you have, for whatever reason, been convinced over the years, just like most everyone else, to regularly and consistently feed your body a diet predominated by food that has had all the life processed or cooked out first.

We humans are unique in that regard. We stand alone as the one and only species in the entire world to remove by cooking what the body needs most from food before we eat it. Then we wonder why we don't feel well. Look at any other species in the natural world, on the land, in the sea, or in the air, and they **all** eat food that has been neither processed nor cooked. And they do not suffer from Fibromyalgia, Lupus, Arthritis, or Chronic Fatigue Syndrome. Or cancer, heart disease, diabetes, osteoporosis, or obesity. **Unless**! Unless they come into contact with us. Animals that are kept in zoos or as pets in our homes or that in some other way have access to what we eat wind up suffering from the very same ailments we suffer from as a result. What does that tell you? How much more obvious could it possibly be?

In one classic, well-known, and highly regarded scientific study that lasted ten years, cats and mice were fed meat and milk and nothing else, no exceptions. The ones fed exclusively raw meat and raw milk **all** lived disease-free until old age. The ones fed exclusively meat and milk cooked and pasteurized **all** suffered numerous diseases and died prematurely.[36] This is a real and well respected study that leaves absolutely no doubt as to what I am saying about living food versus dead food.

The proof of what I am relating to you here about eating food that is living versus food that is not living is verifiable, undeniable, unquestionable, and irrefutable. Yet most people, especially those who are suffering from some form of ill health, eat on average about 10% or **less** living food, and all the rest is non-living food. No wonder they're in pain, sick and out of energy. If you saw someone who bashed himself in the head as hard as he could with a brick four times a day, do you think you would have much difficulty explaining why he always had a headache? Well, that's how obvious the cause of Fibromyalgia, Lupus, Arthritis, and Chronic Fatigue Syndrome is to me when I learn that the sufferer's diet is made up of only 10% living food.

The good news in all of this, in fact the **great** news, is that the dynamic and intelligent living body responds very quickly and effectively when it is simultaneously fed an increased amount of living food and a decreased amount of nonliving food. More people than you might think, who are actively looking for something to help them, immediately make a dramatic change in their diet and start eating far more living food than nonliving food. However it is unrealistic to expect or even suggest that people completely reverse dietary habits that they have had for decades or perhaps their entire life.

Allow me to present to you what is not only realistic but also quite doable and effective. For the sake of discussion, let us suppose that what I am telling you about enzyme-rich living food and overcoming Fibromyalgia, Lupus, Arthritis, and Chronic Fatigue Syndrome is 100% correct. In that case, would it not be **more** than reasonable to recommend that the amount of living food that you eat and the amount of nonliving food you eat be half and half? After all, living food honors and supports the body in all of its activities by using less energy for digestion and producing less waste, whereas nonliving food hinders the body's efforts by using considerably more energy for digestion while giving the body more work to do. That being the case, wouldn't you think that, at the very **least**, half of your food intake should be living regardless of whether you are in a state of good health or not?

I'll take it a step further and say that if you are not willing to assist your body in its efforts by supplying it with a fair share of the living food it requires and craves, then you are probably not serious about your own recovery. Either that or you want to cling to the false hope of some "miracle drug" being discovered that will magically end your Fibromyalgia, Lupus, Arthritis, or Chronic Fatigue Syndrome without having to address their underlying cause.

I am banking on the probability that you are both serious **and** willing to do whatever is necessary to turn this thing around and thus strengthen and energize your body so that your future will be free of Fibromyalgia, Lupus, Arthritis, Chronic Fatigue Syndrome, or any other ailment that is the result of uneliminated toxins.

I know full well that it's one thing to find out and intellectually accept that a genuine and legitimate need exists to feed your body a greater percentage of living food, and it is something else again knowing how to do so sensibly and comfortably. Following this introduction you will find the Three Steps to Recovery. They are designed specifically to help you and guide you through this worthy endeavor. These three steps were not merely slapped together. They are the result of a great deal of study and hands-on experience.

Here's what I can tell you about the Three Steps to Recovery and what you can expect by putting them into practice. I don't want to put castor oil in your tea and tell you it's honey. In other words, I don't want to blue-sky you and make a bunch of wild promises about the level of success you can expect and how quickly they can be expected. I want to be honest and real with you.

Earlier I pointed out that some variables come into play that cannot be explained by anyone, no matter how knowledgeable, no matter how experienced. Different people have different levels of success even though their commitment and effort are the same. There is no accounting for these nondescript variables that operate independently and are unaffected by our actions. Those variables can either work in our favor or not. Haven't we all heard examples of people being told by their doctor that they had only a few months to live who went on to live for years or even decades? Obviously those doctors had no knowledge or control over certain variables for which they could not account.

There are also variables, some very powerful and very influential ones that are **totally within** our control. What I can assure you of is that the Three Steps to Recovery make the very best possible use of them to fully optimize your chances of success. The Three Steps to Recovery are expressly designed to take full advantage of your body's extraordinary recuperative powers. One step is not any more or less important than any other one. It is when all Three Steps are used in unison, as though there were only one step that happened to be divided into three parts, that the greatest results can be expected. As a point of fact, that is exactly the case. It's not as though you do step one and when finished you do step two, finish it, and do step three. All three are undertaken simultaneously. I present them as Three Steps only as a means of describing the process of recovery to you in an understandable way that makes sense and is easy to grasp.

The final determining factor is, of course, your level of commitment and dedication. Obviously, those who halfheartedly dabble with the Three Steps should not expect, nor will they enjoy, nearly the positive results of those who wholeheartedly immerse themselves in them with complete abandon.

The objective of Step One is to jumpstart the process of recovery noticeably. Fibromyalgia, Lupus, Arthritis, and Chronic Fatigue Syndrome are not the beginning stages of the problem but rather the end result of a process that began many years ago. The underlying causes have been at work unchecked for a very long time, and something powerful and dramatic has to be undertaken that will reverse the trend and begin the process of pulling built-up toxins from the connective tissue. Step One definitely achieves that goal.

The purpose of Step Two is to give you a sensible, effective, and yet enjoyable eating lifestyle that not only allows the eating experience to remain a joyous one but also supports the body in all of its healing activities and prevents any further recurrence of symptoms.

Step Three introduces you to a technological breakthrough that turns out to be a Godsend for anyone trying to overcome Fibromyalgia, Lupus, Arthritis, and Chronic Fatigue Syndrome. It is as though it was discovered and developed for the express purpose of fully supporting the goals of the first two steps. In my opinion it is one of, if not the most, important advancements ever made in the area of diet and nutrition. It would not be an exaggeration at all to say that, aside from eating a higher overall amount of living food, the breakthrough to which I am referring will do more to ensure long-term good health than any other factor. That is because it dramatically and significantly improves the effective and efficient digestion of food in the stomach; our highest priority.

My best advice to you is to read the Three Steps with a completely open mind and with the attitude that they are going to be the long sought after answer you have been seeking. Then give them a fair and earnest trial so you will be able to make an accurate assessment of their worth.

CHAPTER FIVE

STEP ONE
TO RECOVERY

Two things have to happen in order for you to both remove the symptoms of Fibromyalgia, Lupus, Arthritis, and Chronic Fatigue Syndrome and to prevent their future return. First, the toxins that are the underlying cause of these ailments and which have overwhelmed the lymph system, causing them to settle in the connective tissue, must be drawn out, broken down, and removed from the body. Second, a manner of eating needs to be adopted that does not overwhelm the lymph system by producing more toxins than it has the ability and energy to eliminate. Step One concerns itself with the first.

We live in a fast-food, quick-fix, I-want-it-right-now world. We want what we want, and we want it **now**. It is that very mentality that the pharmaceutical industry preys upon. People are encouraged and persuaded to take a drug to mask symptoms rather than to address the **cause** of the symptoms and remove them so there would be no need for drugs. There's no money to be made in educating people about how to live in a way that prevents problems before they occur. The life blood of the trillion-dollar drug industry is people who are sick and in pain. You're no good to the drug industry if you are well.

Believe me when I tell you that you did not go to bed healthy one night and wake up in the morning saying, "Oh, darn! I got Fibromyalgia, Lupus, Arthritis, or Chronic Fatigue Syndrome last night." No, no, it takes a very long time to actually reach the point where the lymph system, so capable of handling so much for so long, is in fact overwhelmed to the extent that it can't keep pace and more toxins are generated than eliminated, resulting in their being stored in the tissues.

It is exceedingly important that your mindset isn't one of thinking that all you have to do is change your habits for a little while, get better, and then go back to what you were doing. Rather, the mindset of taking your time and doing it right with permanent changes that result in lifelong well-being, is best.

I cannot impress upon you strongly enough that your number-one consideration should not be how **fast** you are free of symptoms but rather how well you learn how to achieve and **maintain** that desired goal. It doesn't matter if it takes three months or six months or a year or even longer to be completely free of symptoms. What is of greatest importance is that you understand that the very moment you begin to make the principles contained in the Three Steps a permanent part of your lifestyle you have started down a pathway that has but one destination: a life free of pain, whether it be from Fibromyalgia, Lupus, Arthritis, Chronic Fatigue Syndrome, or any other cause. If you stay on that path, no matter what speed you travel, you will ultimately arrive where you want to be; and each step you take brings you one step closer to your goal. Each step you take translates into that much less pain. You're always getting somewhat better and not somewhat worse. Don't rush it. At least you're headed toward your goal and not further from it.

The perfect analogy (have I mentioned that I like analogies?) is if you were driving somewhere in your car. If you should take a wrong turn and go even hundreds of miles away from your intended destination, the **moment** you turn around you are already better off than if you didn't turn around. Every mile you travel in the right direction brings you closer to where you're going.

The same is true with the Three Steps to Recovery. The moment you start using them you have stopped worsening your situation and instead started to improve it. In a relatively short period of time you will start to notice a change, a positive change, in your energy level and all-around well-being.

Okay, so what is the game plan for getting the existing toxins in your body **out**? I have spent considerable time differentiating for you the two primary approaches to eating. One is dominated with foods that have all the life (enzymes) cooked out of them before they are eaten. That way of eating causes the food to stay in the stomach longer, uses far more energy, produces more toxins, gives the lymph system more work to do, and slows the healing process.

The other way of eating is dominated with foods that have **not** had all the life (enzymes) cooked out of them before they are eaten. Those foods require less time in the stomach, require far less energy for digestion, produce fewer toxins, and give the lymph system far less work to do, which thereby speeds up healing. The energy that is not squandered in the stomach unnecessarily by dealing with a prolonged digestive process is automatically made available to the lymph system, which in turn uses it to flush toxins from the body. I have told you throughout that victory over Fibromyalgia, Lupus, Arthritis, and Chronic Fatigue Syndrome will come about as a result of dietetic maneuvering and manipulation. It should therefore come as no surprise to learn that it will be through the use of living food that the symptoms of Fibromyalgia, Lupus, Arthritis, and Chronic Fatigue Syndrome are both removed and prevented from ever returning.

Here's what we know so far:

1. Absolutely every activity of the body requires **some** energy in order to be performed.

2. There is not an unlimited amount of energy available to the body. It has to be replenished every day from the foods we eat.

3. The activity of the body that requires more energy than any other, in fact more than all other activities **combined**, is digestion.

4. The longer food remains in the stomach, the more energy is required and used up, leaving less for use by the lymph system for cleansing and healing.

5. The more efficiently food is digested in the stomach (thereby requiring less energy); the more energy is made available to the lymph system.

6. Nonliving food, that is food that has had its enzymes destroyed by cooking, spends a longer time in the stomach and uses far more energy, depriving the lymph system of the energy it needs.

7. Living food, that is food that has its enzymes intact, spends much less time in the stomach, requires far less energy, and unleashes the healing mechanism of the body (lymph system) by freeing the energy it needs to perform its healing work.

8. As the amount of living food eaten in the diet increases and the amount of the nonliving food simultaneously decreases, the healing activities of the body are enhanced and improved.

Given these facts, it does not take a genius IQ to figure out that the more living food eaten and the less nonliving food eaten, the faster the problems of Fibromyalgia, Lupus, Arthritis, and Chronic Fatigue Syndrome will be overcome.

Interestingly, some people, few in number to be sure, who, upon learning what I have told you so far, actually start to eat **only** living food for as long as it takes to feel completely free of Fibromyalgia, Lupus, Arthritis, and Chronic Fatigue Syndrome. Although I would not try to discourage you from such a severe course of action if you felt you had the discipline to do so, it is not necessary to take such a drastic measure in order to fulfill the objective of Step One. That objective being to significantly lower the level of toxins in your body to a level that is easily manageable by the lymph system.

Many, **many** different ways exist to use living food to achieve any number of health goals, including the lowering of toxins, increasing energy, and ending pain. The method I am going to offer for your consideration is what I call *Mono-Dieting*. A Mono-Diet simply means the eating of **exclusively** living food for a particular length of time, ranging from one day to several months at a time. When Mono-Dieting on exclusively living food, the bare minimum of energy is required for digestion, meaning that a massive amount of energy is freed for use on other activities of the body, primarily that of cleansing and healing.

Most people have never Mono-Dieted even for one day their entire life. Imagine what it must be like when a person's body, accustomed to having the vast majority of available energy directed toward digestion and the rest divided amongst all other activities, has that percentage reversed and a minimum of energy is used in digestion and the bulk is used for cleansing and healing. You may not know what that feels like now, but I can tell you that good things start to happen which are obvious and verifiable. Once you grasp and understand the full magnitude and power inherent in Mono-Dieting, you will, like so many others, come to realize what a potent tool you have for the rest of your life in acquiring and maintaining a high level of pain free good health.

So that there is no question whatever in your mind about what a Mono-Diet is, I want to be absolutely certain you know precisely what it is and how it is utilized. Since a Mono-Diet means eating exclusively living food, let's first make sure you know exactly what comes under the category of a living food.

A living food is one that has not had its enzymes destroyed by heat. A Mono-Diet is eating only fresh, raw, uncooked, and unprocessed foods. Those foods are: fruits, vegetables, their juices, and nuts and seeds. That's it. Nothing else. Let's go over each category one at a time.

Fruit. In terms of our diet, fruit is one of the great gifts of life. The variety from which we can choose is mind-boggling. Most people would be hard-pressed to name 50 different kinds of fruit, but worldwide there are over a 1,000 different kinds of fruit. Few people realize that fruit contains every nutrient (including amino acids to build protein) required by the human species. Plus it contains the finest, purest, and most easily accessible form of energy available from any food. I will discuss the nature of fruit in much greater detail in Step Two, but for now you should know that **any** fruit you are partial to, you should eat. It's not as though one is any better than any other. So whichever ones you are attracted to, have those. **But they must be fresh and uncooked**. No fruit cocktail from a can; it's cooked and dead. No baked, stewed, grilled, or otherwise heated. All are dead. On occasion you will have cooked fruit such as in a baked apple or a piece of pie. I do as well. But **not** when Mono-Dieting. When Mono-Dieting, only living food goes into your living body.

You can eat single pieces of fruit or make fruit salads. Cut up and mix several fruits, make a fruit sauce by pureeing one or more of the fruits, pour it over the top, add a little cinnamon and shredded coconut (raw of course), and you have a beautiful, delicious, healthy, life-giving meal.

Fruits that are a little heavier than the watery fruits, like bananas, raisins, dates, and dried fruit, are also good and work well in fruit salads as well. Plus, they make good, easy-to-carry-around snacks that curb hunger and satisfy the ol' "sweet tooth." One word of caution when eating dried fruit such as figs, prunes, papaya, pineapple, apricots, etc. Make sure they are naturally dried, either sun dried or dried in a dehydrator. Fruit dried with chemicals such as sulpher nitrate is no good. Any health food store will carry naturally dried fruit which tastes far superior and is good for the body instead of hurtful. Also, dried fruit must be eaten sparingly because it is very concentrated. Eat small amounts, or else you will overtax your digestive system, which is exactly what you want to avoid doing.

Special care must also be taken when drinking fruit juices. Depending upon the circumstances under which fruit juices are consumed, they can either be of great benefit to the body and enormously supportive of all of one's health goals, or they can cause great harm and be an underlying hindrance to one's health goals. For fruit juice to be of benefit, it **must** be living, with its enzymes intact, not heated or processed in any way. Something that always rankles me is when supposed "experts" who hold themselves up as authorities make the statement that fruit juices are just as harmful as cola-type soft drinks or any of the other sugary, processed, chemical-laden fruit-flavored drinks that clog the shelves at the grocery store. I am hard-pressed to think of a more imbecilic statement—one that proves without a doubt that perfectly reasonable-appearing people can actually function with a detached brain stem.

I can't help but think that people who dispense such mindless blather have to be proud graduates of one of the medical schools in the United States that does not require a single course on nutrition. These people are so easy to spot. They're usually saying something idiotic like the one about fruit juice, as though they actually knew what they were talking about. I guess they figure that since they earned a Ph.D. in stuffing drugs down the throats of the sick, they can go ahead and make statements on a subject about which they know absolutely nothing, because they made a special point of not studying it for even one hour. What is most exasperating is that unknowing, innocent people take these "experts" seriously. Can you tell that this subject makes the hair stand up on the back of my neck?

If I told you that swimming and drowning were the same thing because they both take place in water, might you think I was just a couple of tweaks away from being confined to the loony bin? When comments about the harmfulness of fruit juice are made, they are done with no distinction whatsoever about the type of fruit juice. The human body must have a certain amount of fat in the diet, or else death would occur. Some vitamins (A, D, E, K) cannot even be utilized unless in the presence of fat. Do you think the fat in a greasy piece of bacon or a deep-fried chicken nugget is the same as the naturally occurring fat found in an avocado or a handful of raw pecans?

All of those multicolored cartons, cans, and bottles of fruit juice that boldly announce their healthy goodness are all pasteurized at a heat so intense that nothing living could survive. All the vitamins, phytonutrients, anti-oxidents, and **enzymes** are destroyed. Many are then treated with synthetic vitamins, additives, food colorings, processed white sugar, and a host of other chemicals, then advertised as something good and wholesome because the word *fruit* is on the label. To compare such a sickening concoction with a fresh-squeezed glass of fruit juice and state that they are both the same because they are chemically similar is naive at best and criminal at worst.

Fresh-squeezed fruit juice, when consumed properly, is a gift from on high. Pasteurized and processed fruit juice is worse than worthless because it acidifies the blood, exacerbates existing conditions such as ulcers, robs the body of essential minerals such as calcium needed to neutralize the acid, and pollutes and overworks the lymph system.

This is no small matter, which is why I am spending time on the subject. As I said, I will be talking about fruit and fruit juice in the next chapter in more detail, but for now, know that the intelligent drinking of fresh-squeezed fruit juice can play an enormous role in your recovery from Fibromyalgia, Lupus, Arthritis, and Chronic Fatigue Syndrome.

By the way, have you ever seen commercials for juicing featuring Jack LaLanne or the Juice Man? These fellows are in their 80s, and they are more vibrant and energetic than many people half their age. Success leaves clues!

Fruit smoothies can also play a huge and significant role during a Mono-Diet. They are delicious, filling, fun, and highly nutritious. A day rarely passes in which I don't have one of these truly delightful treats. A smoothie is made in a blender. Here's my favorite: First you put one or one and a half fresh or frozen bananas in the blender (bananas are frozen by first peeling them, breaking them into pieces and putting them into an airtight container). Add fresh orange juice. Blend them together. Then add any fresh or frozen fruits. I like to add frozen strawberries and blueberries. The more banana you add, the thicker the drink. I also always add a Green Superfood (see chapter eight) to my smoothies. You can make an infinite variety of these smoothies because bananas and a wide variety of frozen fruits are available all year 'round. Experiment with these, and they will quickly become a permanent part of your life, as they have for me.

For those of you whose first reaction to reading this about fruit is to complain that fruit and fruit juices upset your stomach, give you diarrhea, or throw your blood sugar level out of whack, you are soon to learn in the next chapter that there is a right way and a wrong way to consume fruit in terms of the limitations of the human digestive track. Problems such as the ones just mentioned only arise when fruit is eaten incorrectly. Eaten correctly fruit's benefits are unmatched and these problems are avoided.

In addition to fruits (and their juices) the other major component of a Mono-Diet is comprised of veg-etables. And, once again, only fresh and uncooked. Not that vegetables steamed, grilled, sautéed, etc., aren't an extremely important part of a healthy diet; they are, but not when Mono-Dieting. I'm not merely talking about having carrots and celery sticks. I'm talking about having a wide variety of vegetables. I hope you are fond of salads, but if you are one of those people who aren't, you need to be. Salads will play a huge role not only in your recovery from Fibromyalgia, Lupus, Arthritis, and Chronic Fatigue Syndrome but also as an integral part of your eating lifestyle when not Mono-Dieting.

When I talk about a salad, I'm not talking about a wedge of iceberg lettuce with a glop of mayo on it or a few scraps of lettuce with a cherry tomato. I'm talking about a good-sized, full-on, multi-ingredient salad that is interesting, satisfyingly filling, and therefore highly nutritious. Fortunately there are numerous ingredients to choose from and mix and match, so there is no need to be bored with your salads: lettuce (of which there are numerous types) tomatoes, cucumbers, spinach, cabbage, carrots, celery, avocado, sprouts (of which there are many), watercress, radishes, mushrooms, and a host of vegetables that are usually cooked in some manner but can also be eaten raw such as broccoli, cauliflower, beets, corn, green beans and zucchini. I'm not suggesting that all your salads have all these ingredients. You may want a very simple salad of lettuce, tomato, and cucumber. The point is that there are choices you can make so that your salads always remain interesting.

Dressings can also be varied to further the variety and enjoyment of salads. Salads **must** be tasty and interesting, or they will become a chore rather than a delight, so the choice of dressing is an important consideration. This is the one area of Mono-Dieting where there is some leeway with strictness. Many salad dressings, especially creamy ones, aren't 100% uncooked, but the salad itself is so important that some concessions have to be made. Dozens of different salad dressings on the market use high-quality ingredients and have no sugar, additives, preservatives, colorings, or chemicals of any kind, and those are the ones you should seek out. Also, try not to be too heavy-handed with the dressings so the salad isn't "swimming" in dressing.

You can also make a very simple but delicious salad dressing by starting with a high-quality olive oil, add lemon, salt and pepper (if you desire), and herbs and spices. For those of you who like vinegar, let me state that the most widely sold vinegars in supermarkets are a horrendous imitation of the real thing. They are made from coal tar, and there is no place for these rank imposters in a healthy diet. There is one vinegar that is actually beneficial, and it is the only vinegar that you should put into your body. Use only organic, raw, unfiltered, unpasteurized, apple cider vinegar. All health food stores carry Bragg's Organic Apple Cider Vinegar, and that is the one I recommend you use.

Vegetable juices can also be of great benefit when Mono-Dieting. I'm not talking about V-8 juice or other canned juices. They are all pasteurized and worthless. I know they **taste** great, but there are no benefits beyond their taste, and they are in fact counter productive.

Whereas you can certainly find fresh-squeezed orange juice and even fresh juiced apple juice, finding freshly made vegetable juice presents more of a challenge. To have fresh vegetable juice regularly, you might want to think about purchasing a juicer. No matter what the cost, compared to the benefit in terms of improved health that a juicer can bring into your life, it will pay for itself 100 times over.

I don't want to imply that you must have vegetable juice in order to have success in overcoming Fibromyalgia, Lupus, Arthritis, and Chronic Fatigue Syndrome or that a Mono-Diet is not complete without vegetable juices. You can do perfectly well without ever having vegetable juices. But vegetable juices are extremely beneficial, and the point that I am making is that if you do want the added benefit that juices can provide, they **must** be fresh.

I want to urge you in the strongest possible way to seriously consider owning your own personal home juicer for both fruit and vegetable juices. In terms of your health it will be one of the best purchases you ever make.

In my opinion, the best home juicer on the market is the Champion, which I have been using for 30 years. One lasted for 20 years, and I only replaced it because I wanted a different color. The Champion is sturdy, easy to use, and easy to clean. Unlike most juicers that have to be cleaned when the pulp basket inside is full; the Champion can produce an unlimited amount of juice before it needs to be cleaned. That is because both the juice and the pulp are expelled separately simultaneously. Plus, the Champion is less expensive than many juicers of inferior quality.

If you would like more information about the Champion juicer you may call toll-free 877-335-1509 or go to our website: www.fitforlifetime.com.

The only other foods to be eaten when Mono-Dieting besides fruits, vegetables, and their juices are nuts and seeds. I am partial to cashews, almonds, pecans, pumpkin seeds, and sunflower seeds. There are two **extremely** important points that must be made regarding the eating of nuts and seeds. First and foremost is that they have to be raw; not roasted or otherwise heated. When raw, nuts and seeds provide an exceptionally fine source of protein and beneficial fat. When heated they are **highly** acid-forming, take much longer to digest, and toxify and overburden the cleansing mechanism of the body.

The second consideration is that nuts and seeds should be eaten **very** sparingly. They should **not** be overeaten, which is as easy to do as falling off a log. One small handful should do it. They are a very concentrated food that requires far more energy to be digested than fruits and vegetables. Remember, the primary goal of Mono-Dieting is to free energy and conserve it whenever possible. The ideal time to have a small amount of nuts and seeds is about 3:00 or so in the afternoon when you might be feeling hungry because lunch was three hours earlier and dinner might not be for three hours later. Nuts and seeds stay in the stomach longer and take away those hunger pangs. But be very careful with nuts and seeds. Eating them every day and filling up on them defeats the very purpose of Mono-Dieting, which is to free energy for the lymph system to remove toxins from the body.

As an aside, I will tell you that whenever I have nuts and seeds, I always like to have slices of cucumber with them. It tastes great, and the water content of the less concentrated cucumbers seems to help move the nuts and seeds through the stomach more quickly and efficiently. Give it a try. It's very tasty and satisfying.

Now that you know what foods are ideal for a Mono-Diet, the most obvious and logical question is, "What is the duration and frequency of a Mono-Diet? How long do they last, and how often are they undertaken?"

A Mono-Diet can be as short as one day or last as long as several months. In terms of getting a handle on

Fibromyalgia, Lupus, Arthritis, and Chronic Fatigue Syndrome, the purpose of Mono-Dieting is to draw out toxins from the connective tissue that have been accumulating there for who knows how long. This is goal one. No matter what other measures are taken to reduce the overall production of toxins or to prevent the further buildup of toxins in the tissues, no real progress will be made and no lasting relief of symptoms will be realized until the existing built-up toxins, which are the underlying cause of the problem, are removed. That is the goal **and** the result of well planned and conducted Mono-Diets.

Over the next six months, I am going to ask you to go on six Mono-Diets: one week out of each month. Now please don't jump to the conclusion that, because I'm saying six months, that's how long you are going to have to wait in order to start to feel better. Remember what I shared with you earlier about certain nondescript variables that come into play and which effect how quickly different people start to feel relief. Some people will feel considerably better in as little as two months or less, while for others, under the same circumstances, it can be as much as six months or more. That's just how it is, and the only way to find out which group you are in is to go through the process. Obviously, it is my wish that everyone will see marked improvement in record time, but experience has shown me that the times necessary for improvement vary from person to person.

Also, remember this: The moment you start, you will begin to see **some** improvement. And no matter how small that improvement may be at first, it's a far sight better than **no** improvement at all or, worse yet, a further worsening of the condition. Recall, if you will, the analogy of taking a wrong turn in your car and traveling far out of your way. The moment you turn your car around and head in the right direction you stop compounding your mistake, and every mile takes you closer to your goal.

For the sake of understanding, from here on out, let's refer to the way you will be eating as either being on a *Mono-Diet* or on your **regular diet**. For the next six months I'm asking you to go on a one-week Mono-Diet followed by three weeks on your regular diet. During the one-week Mono-Diet, nothing, but **nothing**, goes into your body that has been cooked, heated, or processed in any way. Even if you are one of the majority of people who feel very much better in a shorter rather than longer time, stick with it and do the full six months. It is literally impossible to Mono-Diet too much, but you can definitely Mono-Diet too little in order to fully get the job done. You can be certain, without a doubt, that it took far longer than six months to create the problem of Fibromyalgia, Lupus, Arthritis, or Chronic Fatigue Syndrome in the first place, so if they can be significantly and demonstrably improved in six months, that's a pretty good deal, don't you think?

Undoubtedly, there will be those who have suffered long and who are therefore eager to accelerate the process of cleansing by Mono-Dieting more frequently and for a longer duration than one week out of each month. One of the great advantages of Mono-Dieting is its great versatility. It can be utilized in so many different ways. No hard and fast rules exist that must be adhered to at all costs regarding length and frequency of Mono-Dieting. Of course, in order for Step One to be successful, each month of the next six months must have seven **consecutive** days of Mono-Dieting, but other than that you can Mono-Diet as much or as little as you wish in addition to the seven consecutive days.

For example, instead of a Mono-Diet of one week and a regular diet for three weeks, you can Mono-Diet for one week and regular diet for only two weeks. Or, if you are really gung ho, you can Mono-Diet every other week interspersed with every other week on your regular diet. Or you can Mono-Diet two or three days during the weeks of regular dieting. Or maybe one month you Mono-Diet for the one week and another month you Mono-Diet for two weeks. The point that I am making is that you can Mono-Diet for any number of days or weeks you want, anytime you want, and in any order you want, just so long as during each of the next six months there are at **least** seven consecutive days of Mono-Dieting. Also, even if you Mono-Diet more than the minimum of one week a month, do so for the full six months. In other words, if you Mono-Diet for two weeks a month instead of one, you still do it for six months, not three months.

I know this calls for a significant commitment on your part, but what I want, and what you should want, is to do the job right and do it right the first time. Six months may appear now to be a long time to strictly adhere to seven consecutive days of Mono-Dieting out of each month, but I am interested in your feeling good, being energetic, free of pain, and off drugs six **years** from now, **26** years from now. The first six months are crucial to that goal. Give it your full and dedicated commitment now, when it is so important that you do so, and you will be glad for the rest of your life.

There are two cautionary pieces of advice that I need to bring to your attention. The first has to do with the manner in which you eat when you end your seven-day Mono-Diets and return to your regular diet. The tendency is to end the seven days and go on an eating rampage and eat all the foods you have been missing and dreaming about for a week. I'll tell you the truth; it's what most people do even when warned against such a course of action. In the past I have done it myself, even though I, of all people, know better. It's a destructive act that counteracts much of the good accomplished during the Mono-Diet. It catches the body off guard, so to speak, and can throw it into turmoil. The best advice I can give you is to go slowly the first couple of days after a one-week Mono-Diet. Don't overeat, and don't have **all** the favorites you have been craving the very first day.

The second possibility I need to discuss with you is an enormously important one that you **must** be mindful of so you will know how to handle it properly should it occur. What I'm referring to is the fact that occasionally—and I want to emphasize that it doesn't always happen, but only occasionally—the very symptoms of pain and lethargy that an effort is being made to overcome first become more intensified. As I said, it doesn't happen to everyone, and happens only on occasion, but it is a real possibility, especially for those people who are the most toxic and whose bodies are in the greatest need of a thorough cleansing.

I know that the idea of making a dramatic and committed effort to remove the symptoms of Fibromyalgia, Lupus, Arthritis, and Chronic Fatigue Syndrome that results instead in a **worsening** of the symptoms is not a very pleasant prospect, but sometimes it is a necessary one. Never lose sight of the fact that your living body is **always** on the lookout for ways to cleanse itself and heal itself. When, all of a sudden, after many years, a tremendous amount of energy is freed, which is exactly what happens when Mono-Dieting, the body rushes to remove toxins as quickly as possible, not knowing if it will have another opportunity. This is, of course, why symptoms initially intensify. But as soon as the body acclimates itself to the regular supply of energy, the symptoms will start to subside.

It is understandable if the initial response to a worsening of symptoms while Mono-Dieting elicits something to the effect of, "Hey, this stinks! I was better off before, **without** this brilliant idea." If it should turn out that you are one of those to whom this does happen, be uplifted and encouraged by the fact that it is a clear statement that the integrity of the healing mechanism in your body is intact and functioning well. It may be temporarily uncomfortable, but you are witnessing healing in action. It's a good thing, not a bad thing. It shows, in no uncertain terms, that your journey of recovery has begun.

I can tell you, from 35 years of experience, that it will pass, so the absolute, most damaging thing you can possibly do is stop the process of healing and return to your old way of eating and taking drugs to mask the symptoms. You would be better off not to start in the first place than to actually get to the point where your body begins the healing process only to have the door slammed in its face. Have faith that your body knows what it's doing. Stay the course and see it through. The discomfort will pass. It always does.

One further point of importance needs to be made here. After you have completed the initial six months, wherein you Mono-Diet at least one week out of each month, it would serve you well to Mono-Diet periodically thereafter. If you Mono-Dieted two, three, or four times a year—meaning a week every few months or so—it would be of immeasurable help to your body in staying on top of things. Also, one or even two days a week on all living food has enormous benefit as well. My point is for you not to abandon Mono-Dieting after the first six months just because you are feeling better. It is a lifelong tool that should be used as preventative maintenance. You cannot Mono-Diet too much, only too little. Prioritize it. Fit it into your lifestyle the way you would anything else of extreme importance and value.

Perhaps right now, when Mono-Dieting is so new to you, there's some uneasiness about it all. But, I assure you, once you are more familiar with it and get the hang of it, you will see how sensible and worthwhile it is. You just have to start. Imagine how confusing it is for someone the very first time s/he sits down at a piano, having never taken a lesson. All those keys. But after learning the different keys and practicing how to play, the confusion goes away, and the more s/he practices the better s/he becomes. **Understanding comes through doing.**

Now that you know what Step One is—Mono-Dieting for at least one week each month over the next six months—the most logical next question would have to be, "How do I eat during the six months when not Mono-Dieting, and how do I eat after the first six months?" That is the subject of Step Two to Recovery.

CHAPTER SIX

STEP TWO
TO RECOVERY

You have learned how vitally important it is to Mono-Diet in order to pull out the built-up toxins in the connective tissue that cause the symptoms of Fibromyalgia, Lupus, Arthritis, and Chronic Fatigue Syndrome and flush them from the body. It is equally important, and every bit as crucial, to eat in such a manner when not Mono-Dieting so as to fully support and further the goals you are wishing to achieve and which Mono-Dieting helps you achieve.

It would make no sense whatsoever to make the effort necessary to unleash the powerful cleansing and healing mechanism of your body only to return to the very manner of eating that brought on the problem in the first place. Could you imagine someone's going through a 12-Step Program to overcome alcoholism and then celebrating by getting drunk?

I'm going to be recommending you make two dietary changes that are probably quite different from what you are presently doing. They are not complicated, they are not difficult to implement, and they are not going to put you through some complex undertaking that turns the eating experience into an ordeal and ultimately leaves you hungry and craving all the time. They are only **different**. You will still get to eat the foods you like. You will not have to carry around a calculator and a measuring cup. You will not have to go hungry. You will be able to eat until satisfied. You will be able to eat out at restaurants. It is a way of eating that not only fulfills your desire to eat and eat well but also honors the body's digestive limitations and provides the energy necessary for ongoing cleansing and healing.

A most interesting attribute of human beings, one that seems to be intrinsically encoded into our genetic makeup, is our never ending desire for change. We want what's new, better, different, revolutionary, innovative, and novel. We want the newest model, the latest edition, the most up-to-date improvement. We want what's avant-garde and ultramodern. We want the state-of-the-art, latest and greatest of everything and anything under the sun. And we want it **now**! That's why you can go to the store and buy the latest version of a computer and by the time you get it home and hooked up, it's already obsolete.

Imagine how unbearably monotonous life would become if, from this point on, nothing in any area of life changed. Nothing new was ever designed or improved upon. Whether it was cars, fashion, computers, politics, social issues, sports, business ventures— you name it—what if **nothing** changed or was improved or was different in any way. We would start to see obituaries with cause of death listed as "acute intolerable boredom."

One old expression says it well: "The only thing constant in this world is change." And that is life as we know it today. Nothing stays the same. Knowing that to be so, what certainly has to be tops on the list in the Irony Hall of Fame is the one area of life that has had little or no change for at least 100 years. I say it is ironic because it is an area of far greater importance than if hemlines will be above or below the knee, if cars will go faster on less fuel, or if computers will have greater gigabyte capacity.

The area to which I am referring, you have probably guessed, is our basic approach toward eating. Essentially, it's a hearty breakfast in the morning and meat and potatoes for dinner. It's been that way for all of my 60 years. How about you? I'd say the most notable change in dietary recommendations that has come from the scientific community was when the four food group circle was changed to the four food group pyramid. I'm not suggesting that no changes have been made. People are trying to eat more fiber in their diet and are making an attempt to ingest less salt, cholesterol, and fried foods, but fundamentally it's all within the context of a hearty breakfast and meat and potatoes.

Don't you think some innovative changes should also be made in the area of life that keeps us **alive**? Why would this be the one area not to change? Especially when one considers that more people, **including children**, are overweight now than at any other time in history. Catastrophic diseases such as heart disease, cancer, diabetes, osteoporosis, and obesity have been rising steadily for decades. And, of course, so have Fibromyalgia, Lupus, Arthritis, and Chronic Fatigue Syndrome. We are in the midst of an explosion of McFast food which is taking its toll on our most precious of treasures: our children. Did you know that over 90% of the children in the United States have at least one symptom of heart disease?[37] It's shameful. The approach toward eating that has been in effect for so long is in dire need of an overhaul, and the time for it is right now.

In August 2003, the **Washington Post** ran a story wherein it stated that, "The latest indication of a deepening health crisis because of the nation's obesity epidemic. ..." is the fact that "the number of overweight children tripled between 1970 and 2000."[38] Now the question we should all be asking is: What advice have we been following during these 30 years to cause an "obesity epidemic" during which time childhood obesity has tripled, and who has been giving the advice? The answer is that we have been following the advice to eat a hearty breakfast and to adhere to the meat-and-potato concept. And who has given this advice that has obviously not worked and put us into this dire situation? Medical doctors and their allies, the American Dietetic Association.

Medical doctors who know little or nothing about nutrition either give advice anyway or advise patients to find a Registered Dietitian to help them. Many registered Dietitians are woefully behind the times in terms of what constitutes proper nutrition and advise patients to listen to their doctors. A cozy little setup that has resulted in the most dire overweight epidemic in history. The proof is in. The evidence is clear and could not possibly be more obvious. The advice has been wrong, dead wrong, and we must **stop** listening to these people on matters of proper diet.

You will be pleased to learn that the Three Steps to Recovery that you will be following to overcome Fibromyalgia, Lupus, Arthritis, and Chronic Fatigue Syndrome will also normalize your body weight. You won't have to do anything more in order to lose weight if you need to. In the process of the body's "fixing" itself, it will automatically shed excess weight.

As is usually the case whenever something new comes along that upsets established, conventional thinking, it is initially met with resistance. Arthur Schoepenhauer put it best in one of his most notable quotes: "All truth goes through three stages. First it is ridiculed. Then it is violently opposed. Finally it is accepted as self-evident."

I am not so naïve as to think I will escape the ire of those who have a vested interest in things staying just the way they are. The fact is, I welcome any fair and true scrutiny of the dietary changes I suggest. I think healthy skepticism is appropriate and weeds out that which cannot stand the test of time. My problem is with the type of out-of-hand rejection without honest investigation, which has become so predictable from those "experts" who have made a point of not studying nutrition or those who have, such as Registered Dietitians, who know a whole lot about what is not so.

Anyone who conducts even a cursory study of the American Dietetic Association quickly learns that it thrives on corporate cash and therefore kowtows to big industry interests. The American Dietetic Association is in the business of maintaining the status quo and will attack anyone who does not toe the party line. It's almost as though their primary objective is to undermine anything new and innovative that ultimately might prove how little the Association actually knows about proper nutrition.

Fortunately, the dietary changes I am about to suggest to you **have** withstood the test of time. Plus, they are exceedingly easy to verify for oneself. In literally less than two weeks' time they reveal themselves to be the boon I am suggesting they are. I openly welcome and encourage anyone to put them to the most rigid of tests, because I know from experience that the more they are scrutinized, the more they prove their worth and value.

As I have stated, the two most counterproductive yet persistently lingering customs of the standard American diet (SAD) are the belief in the importance of a "hearty" breakfast and the habit of combining different types of foods at a single meal—known as the "meat-and-potato" concept. These are the two areas in which changes need to be made, and when they **are** made, changes in your health quickly follow.

The first recommendation I wish to present to you concerns itself with what is or is not the most healthy breakfast. What foods eaten in the early morning hours support the goal and further the effort to cleanse body tissues of toxins while providing the body with the optimum amount of nutrition and energy?

In order to present what may be a brand-new concept to you in a way that is sensible, logical, understandable, and which appeals to your common sense, I want to bring your attention back to the very opening of the book. I was talking about the grandeur and splendor of life in all its magnificence. The point was made that three fundamental activities must be present in order for life to exist. Do you remember what they are? First, there must be some means of taking in nutrition. Second, there must be some form of metabolism to extract those nutrients. Third, there must be some capacity to eliminate wastes.

Are you familiar with the terms *Circadian Rhythms, Biological Clock*, or *Body Cycles*? All three refer to well defined, regularly recurring cycles of biological activities in the human body that occur in certain set intervals every 24 hours. In what most assuredly stands as a stunning testimony to the synergy, harmony, and interconnectedness of all the biological factors that govern our existence, there exists three eight-hour cycles of the human body that just so happen to coincide **exactly** with the three fundamental activities of life.

The eight-hour body cycle that coincides with the taking in of nutrition is called the *Appropriation Cycle*. It extends from 12 noon until 8 PM and it is the time when the body is most predisposed to taking in food. The eight-hour body cycle that coincides with metabolism and the extraction of nutrients is called the *Assimilation Cycle*. It extends from 8 PM until 4 AM, and it is when the body is extracting and absorbing nutrients. The eight-hour body cycle that coincides with the elimination of wastes is called the *Elimination Cycle*. It extends from 4 AM until 12 noon, and it is when the eliminative faculties of the body are at their most heightened.

It's rather obvious when you think about it: We eat (Appropriation), we extract what we need from the food (Assimilation), and we get rid of what's left (Elimination). The cycle of greatest concern, in terms of eliminating the toxins that can cause the symptoms of Fibromyalgia, Lupus, Arthritis, and Chronic Fatigue Syndrome, is the Elimination Cycle. This is the one that must be focused upon. **Any** measure that can be taken that streamlines and improves the Elimination Cycle must be nurtured. And any practice that hinders or retards the Elimination Cycle must be discontinued. **This is the key to your success**—an Elimination Cycle that is in no way hindered or prevented from performing its duties with the highest possible efficiency.

I want to clarify two points before continuing, to remove all confusion. First, elimination of wastes does not refer solely to a bowel movement. Although bowel movements certainly are a primary means of removing waste from the body, the Elimination Cycle is involved in the gathering of waste that is produced by every one of the some 100 trillion cells of the body. Some of this waste will undoubtedly be removed through the bowels, but waste is also removed from the bladder, skin, and with every breath that is exhaled.

Second, when I refer to the Elimination Cycle, which goes from 4 AM until 12 noon, that does not mean that at 4 AM sharp the Elimination Cycle fires up and at the stroke of 12 noon it shuts down. The elimination of wastes from the body is so exceedingly crucial to life itself that it is a process that is ongoing, to some degree, at all times (as are all the cycles). During the hours of 4 AM until 12 noon the degree of intensity is at its very highest. At no other time is it higher, only lower. And it is the degree of intensity of the Elimination Cycle that is of greatest importance.

It's a simple equation. Every activity of the body requires some energy. Since there is only a set amount of energy available for use by the body each day, the more activities there are using that energy, the less there will be for each one. It can be compared to taking money from a bank account to pay bills. If there is more money in the account than there are bills, then they can all be paid, no problem. But if there is **less** money than there are bills, only some can be paid until more money is deposited into the account.

One factor exists that, more than any other, increases the intensity of the Elimination Cycle. It is when the digestive process, which as you know requires more energy than anything else, is at rest. When no digestion is going on in the stomach, the Elimination Cycle has all the energy it needs. As soon as food enters the stomach, a significant amount of the energy is diverted from Elimination for use in digestion.

People have been trained and conditioned like Pavlov's dogs to awaken in the morning and eat a "hearty breakfast." And that, dear reader, is when all the trouble starts. Let's say, for example, that you wake up in the morning at 7 AM or 8 AM and have breakfast. That is right smack in the middle of the Elimination Cycle (4 AM till 12 noon), when its efforts are at the absolute highest. Firing up the digestive process at that time puts a strangle hold on the Elimination Cycle.

To me it is a tragedy that there are people whose Elimination Cycle has never ever, even for one day of their life, been allowed to function uninterrupted from 4 AM until 12 noon. I know some of you right now are saying, "Hey, **I'm** one of those people." And I'm telling you that that is a primary reason why you are dealing with Fibromyalgia, Lupus, Arthritis, or Chronic Fatigue Syndrome.

So the first of the two dietary changes I am suggesting you make is that you do not eat anything that requires digestion in the stomach from the time you awaken in the morning until at least 12 noon. This will undoubtedly be the biggest challenge for those who love eating a traditional breakfast. But, be clear, I'm not saying not to eat **anything** for breakfast. I'm saying not to eat anything that must digest in the stomach. And before I describe to you what foods **do not** digest in the stomach and therefore do not diminish the efforts of the Elimination Cycle in any way, I must address the most common and yet at the same time most illogical and baseless comment ever associated with the debate over eating breakfast.

"You have to eat a good, hearty breakfast for energy." Have you ever heard that one? It's usually the advice that comes from the people who "don't know" or from dietitians who think they do. It is extremely important that you fully and truly understand, without any doubt, what a ridiculously absurd statement that is. You don't feel energized after eating, you feel tired. And the bigger the meal, the more tired you are. That's because it **requires** energy, and a good deal of it, to digest food. This is totally self-evident. You don't need a scientist or a scientific study to tell you if you're tired or not.

The process of transforming food into energy takes a long time—hours. And what is ironic is that the process (like **all** activities of the body) **takes** energy to be completed. That is why most of the energy you will have for use during the day is built up while you are asleep and the body's activities are at its lowest. Waking up in the morning with the full complement of energy for the day and spending a big chunk of it on a meal doesn't **give** you energy, it **uses** energy. What do you think that midmorning slump is all about that prompts all those cups of coffee for the caffeine lift?

If I told you that the gas tank in my car wasn't quite full, so I was going to drive the car around the block a few dozen times to fill it to the top, you would start to have doubts about my sanity. Yet some psuedoscientist in a white smock can say something equally as loopy, and it's taken seriously.

Now I know that some of you may be thinking that the energy from breakfast will be available later in the day if not immediately following the meal. That seems reasonable, and is certainly what some ill-informed dietitians will tell you. But, once again, that is faulty thinking. Follow me here, and you'll see why. Let's say you wake up in the morning and have a traditional breakfast. That food will be in the stomach for at **least** three hours before it enters the intestines and the job of transforming the food into energy can even begin. Before that process can be completed, it's lunchtime! Another meal enters the stomach for its three-hour stay before entering the intestines. And before the process of turning it into energy can be completed, it's dinner-time! Get the picture?

You don't become more energetic as the day unfolds; it's just the opposite. When you finally go to bed at night it is because you're **tired**, not because you're bouncing off the walls with energy. It is during your sleep that your body finally has the opportunity to build up your energy supply. Eating a hearty breakfast for energy is complete nonsense, promoted by the ill-informed and big business.

The one exception to all of this is, of course, when breakfast consists of the one food in existence that does **not** require any digestive energy in the stomach and therefore does not hinder the Elimination Cycle in any way. It passes through the stomach relatively quickly and is broken down in the intestines, where it does indeed turn into available energy in less than an hour. The food to which I'm referring is....fruit. Unlike any other food you eat, no matter what it is, fruit requires **no** digestion in the stomach.

Let me be crystal clear here so there is no doubt about what I am recommending. From the time you awaken in the morning until at least 12 noon, you eat absolutely nothing other than fruit. Not a single bite of toast. Not a teaspoon of cottage cheese. Nothing but fruit, fruit salad, fruit juice, or fruit smoothies. As much as you desire. Some people can have a glass of orange juice and a banana and not want anything more until lunchtime. Others want to have some grapes or a peach or an apple every hour. No problem. You can have as much or as little as it takes to see you through until noon. And don't forget, whatever you have **must** be fresh and unpasteurized, or else the purpose is defeated.

Some people will easily be able to make this transition because they weren't all that interested in eating breakfast in the first place and only did so because they were misled into thinking that it was a healthful practice. For others, it will be a greater challenge, and they may very well be saying to me right now, "No breakfast?! You can go to where the fires never go out." But I will tell you this: It may be a big challenge to go from a heavy, bacon-and-egg breakfast to one of only fruit, but the habit of doing so will bring you greater rewards than any other dietary practice you could undertake. I know what a brazen statement that is, but it is not made in haste, and it is one that is backed up by the results of literally hundreds of thousands of people, if not millions, over the last quarter of a century.

Over the years, thanks to the success and popularity of **FIT FOR LIFE**, I have been interviewed in all areas of the media more times than I can recall. For some reason, one of the most frequent questions asked of me is, after studying diet and nutrition for so many years, what principle do I consider to be the single most important and valuable one I have ever learned? No question could be answered more easily. The principle of eating exclusively fruit till noon is undoubtedly the most important piece of knowledge I have ever learned in my 35 years of study, and I thank God every day that its importance was brought to my attention. I know that it, more than any other factor, is responsible for my recovery from some very debilitating and painful conditions. And it remains today as the foundation stone for why I am able to live a healthy existence in spite of my challenges with Agent Orange poisoning.

If you take one thing and nothing else from this book, make it the understanding of the importance of eating exclusively fruit till noon so that your Elimination Cycle is allowed to proceed unfettered. If you do that and nothing else, you will see a marked improvement in your symptoms of Fibromyalgia, Lupus, Arthritis, and Chronic Fatigue Syndrome.

Since the first **FIT FOR LIFE** book was written in 1985, I have received over half a million letters from people commenting on one aspect or another of what the book did for them. I could write a complete book on the comments alone pertaining to the effects of eating fruit till noon. In fact, there were more comments about the positive effects of eating fruit till noon than all other comments **combined**. To this day, people contact me by mail or fax or e-mail or by stopping me on the street to tell me that it is the one principle they stick to no matter what, because it has changed their life. They have more energy, more vitality, less pain and ill health, and it has become their greatest ally in acquiring and maintaining a high level of good health.

Some people are literally brought to tears when they tell me of the way it has rescued them from problems that tormented them for years. Invariably they say that before making fruit till noon a permanent part of their lifestyle and actually experiencing the good it produces, they would never have believed that so much good could come from one simple change in their eating habits.

Most of the comments refer to the astonishing difference in their energy levels but it is the way that it has effected their life overall that impresses them most. Whatever else you may or may not do in your quest to overcome Fibromyalgia, Lupus, Arthritis, and Chronic Fatigue Syndrome, I hope for your sake that you fully explore the possibilities of what you can experience by allowing your Elimination Cycle to function fully and unhindered as a result of correctly eating only fruit till noon.

I told you earlier that it proves itself to anyone willing to give it a fair trial, so here is what I suggest you do. Start tomorrow morning to eat only fruit from the time you wake up until 12 noon. Do it for one week without making any other dietary changes, so you will be able to be certain that anything you feel is because of eating only fruit in the morning. On the eighth day have whatever type of traditional breakfast you were having before this test. Try to work it out so the eighth day falls on a weekend. You'll need to rest. Millions of people have taken this challenge and have had their mind blown, and you can as well. The difference is obvious and unmistakable.

If the concept of eating only fruit till noon is brand-new to you and a breakfast of traditional foods such as pancakes or bacon and eggs or oatmeal or some boxed breakfast cereal with milk is something you look forward to and enjoy, you may have difficulty believing my next statement. The longer you eat only fruit till noon, the easier and more natural it becomes. Since an unobstructed Elimination Cycle is in tune with the physiological body cycles, the body itself becomes accustomed to the practice of fruit till noon.

Believe it or not, a time will come a time when the mere **thought** of eating a heavy, non-fruit breakfast will become objectionable to you. I know people personally who have told me that because I was so convincing and it made so much sense intellectually and the need for relief from painful symptoms so strong that they would start eating only fruit till noon and stick to it for as long as need be. But they would never stop craving the old traditional breakfasts, no matter how good they felt. These same people have, almost sheepishly, acknowledged to me that they were stunned at how fanatical they had become about fruit till noon and how little desire they had for the "old way" of eating breakfast.

In one case, a very famous athlete whose name you would immediately recognize but I am not at liberty to reveal, became so enamored with eating only fruit till noon that he had a standing rule in his house saying that whether you were into **FIT FOR LIFE** or not, nothing but fruit or fruit juice would be eaten in his house before noon.

Having only fruit till noon is not something to do until you are healed of whatever ailment you are wrestling with only to return to the old way of eating down the line. It is a lifelong commitment. Now that is not to say that on occasion you will not have breakfast foods other than fruit. And, quite frankly, there's nothing wrong with that if it's something you want to do. It's what you do most of the time that counts, and aside from a noticeable lack of energy on those days, having a big breakfast once in a while is not going to harm you in any way. When you do it, enjoy it and refrain from feeling guilty or browbeating yourself. The fact is, the way you feel on those days will keep you from doing it with any regularity.

It's essential that this way of eating be a lifestyle that ebbs and flows freely without absolute rules and regulations that must be adhered to at all costs. I will say this, however. During the first six months when you are Mono-Dieting one week out of each month, the best can be expected if your breakfasts were consistently comprised exclusively of fruit.

In order to help you have a greater understanding of the unique nature of fruit and the optimum manner in which it should be consumed, I'm going to give you a few helpful hints to assist you.

You have learned that fruit is the one food in the human diet that does not require any digestion in the stomach. Because of that fact, fruit (which includes fruit juice and fruit smoothies) should be consumed only on an empty stomach, not with or immediately following any other food. In this country eating fruit as a dessert is a way of life. If you eat fruit with or immediately following foods that must stay in the stomach (which are **all** foods other than fruit), bad things happen.

The human body's bloodstream is slightly alkaline and must remain so to maintain good health. The more acidic the diet, the more problems result. Fruit is alkaline and is instrumental in maintaining the body's acid/alkaline pH balance. When fruit is forced to be in the stomach with foods that are being digested there, the fruit, which is alkaline, instantly turns acidic. This can cause, or aggravate, existing ulcers, bring on stomachaches, and cause all the food in the stomach to spoil.

Some people complain that they can't eat melon or strawberries or oranges, and that is because they are eaten **after** a meal and thereby ferment, turn to acid, and cause stomach problems. This is invariably blamed on the fruit. When these and other fruits are eaten correctly, meaning **before** other foods, they pass through the stomach without any problems. If you are one of those people who experience pain and discomfort after eating fruit, simply try eating it alone and on an empty stomach, and you will see for yourself what a difference it makes.

Many people don't eat what are referred to as the "acid fruits" such as oranges, grapefruit, and pineapples because of the very problem stated above. After eating or drinking the juices of these fruits, their stomach hurts. But their classification as acid fruits is only a botanical classification. **All** fruit inside the body is alkaline **unless** it is heated, eaten with or following other foods, or its juices are pasteurized. Then it is highly acidic and harmful. You are much better off drinking water or nothing at all rather than drinking pasteurized orange juice, which is the type of orange juice most people drink. That includes juices made from concentrate, all of which are pasteurized.

While we're on the subject of drinking juice, it is important to note that juice should not be gulped down. When you drink juice, drink it slowly. One mouthful at a time so it can mix with saliva and not overwhelm the stomach. This is no small issue. It may not seem like a big deal, but it is. Always drink your juices slowly.

I would say that the number-one benefit of **correctly** eating fruit is the energy that it produces. You may or may not be aware of it, but the human brain can burn one thing and one thing only for fuel: sugar in the form of glucose. It cannot burn protein directly, it cannot burn fat directly, and it cannot burn starch directly. Absolutely everything that is eaten has to ultimately be turned to glucose first before it can be used. Although the body **can** turn protein and fat into glucose, it is an extremely complex and energy-intensive process compared to the ease with which it turns carbohydrates to glucose. Guess what? The sugar component in fruit (fructose) turns to glucose faster and with greater ease than anything else in the human diet other than mother's milk. When eaten **correctly** it can be in the bloodstream as utilizable energy for the brain in less than one hour. Everything else takes four or five times that long. That's why so many people who start to eat fruit correctly and eat it exclusively from the time they waken in the morning until 12 noon rave about the increase in their energy level.

In the previous chapter I mentioned that people sometimes express concern about eating more fruit and the effect it will have on their blood sugar level. Eating fruit **correctly** will help stabilize the blood sugar level. One can't have low blood sugar when there is plenty of sugar in the blood. Not the refined, processed sugar that dominates the American diet and is a poison as far as the living body is concerned. That sugar will most definitely cause significant problems. The truly natural sugar obtained from fresh, wholesome fruit, **properly eaten**, cause none of the problems associated with one's blood sugar level.

The same holds true for fruit sugar causing or contributing to diabetes. Now here's an interesting tidbit about which the vast majority of people are ill informed: diabetes is **not** caused by the consumption of too much sugar. Diabetes is caused by the overconsumption of fat which destroys the insulin producing glands in the pancreas. Once those glands are rendered useless and insulin is not available to metabolize sugar, diabetes results. Unfortunately people jump to the completely erroneous conclusion that it is sugar that causes the problem in the first place. It would not surprise me in the least if I were to learn that a few years down the line, in addition to an increased incidence of heart disease and cancer, there was a striking increase as well in the incidence of diabetes as a result of so many unfortunate people being deceived into going on those all-protein or high-protein diets.

For those of you who have diabetes and want to try these recommendations what I can tell you honestly is this: Of all the maladies that can occur in human beings, diabetes is without a doubt the most trouble-some and challenging due to the numerous unknown variables that can come into play. What I can tell you is that some people with diabetes have done very well following the **FIT FOR LIFE** recommendations, including the eating of fruit, and others have not. I wish I knew the answer to why that is but I don't. All you can do is follow the recommendations while keep-ing a close eye on your condition and see which cate-gory you are in. I wish I had something more to offer but diabetes has been a great enigma for me and the scientific community for decades. I have noticed that those on oral medication versus injections have an eas-ier time of it but both have some success.

Considering that fruit fulfills the requirement for nutrients and energy more fully and perfectly than any other food in the human diet when eaten correctly, is it not peculiar that fruit is relegated to the last place on the menu as almost an afterthought, and is all too often used merely for ornamental purposes?

I wish to revisit for just a moment the subject dis-cussed in the introduction to the Three Steps to Recovery pertaining to the comment that all sugar is the same in the body, whether it's from a candy bar or a fresh peach. Because of uninformed statements like that, people have been frightened into thinking that eating as much fruit as I am suggesting will make them fat. That is true only when fruit is eaten **incorrectly**—in other words, when it is heated, or eaten with or immediately following other foods. When fruit is eaten correctly, not only will it not make you fat but it will help you **lose** weight.

It's important that you understand that eating fruit till noon does not mean that at 12 noon you must have something other than fruit or that you must have a meal at all. Fruit till noon means at **least** until noon. If you are not hungry, or if you want to continue having fruit until dinnertime, that's perfectly fine. On occasion you simply won't feel like eating—not fruit, not anything, and that's fine. Or you may want to have fruit later in the day as a snack or later at night, which is also fine. But one super important point must be kept in mind. Although fruit can be eaten 20 to 30 minutes **before** any other food, once anything other than fruit has been eaten, at **least** three hours must elapse before eating fruit again. This is exceedingly important. If you wish to have fruit or juice after lunch or after dinner at night, be sure it has been three hours since the meal.

Bananas, raisins, dates, and dried fruit are more concentrated than watery fruits (apples, oranges, grapes, melons, etc.), so they give you a more "full" feeling when eating only fruit till noon. They also make great snacks as long as it's been three hours since eating anything other than fruit.

Finally, I want to remind you that when taking the seven-day test of fruit till noon, the possibility exists of your feeling out of sorts the first two or three days. You could feel stuffed up or lethargic or edgy for no apparent reason or even have a minor bout of diarrhea. As I said earlier when discussing this very possibility, most people do not experience any of these effects. But if you should, realize that the dynamic body suddenly has newfound available energy to work with and it is initiating a cleansing. It's not the fun part, I know. However, it is necessary, and it is beneficial. Hang in there.

Now to the second dietary change I will be asking of you—the one associated with meat and potatoes. It concerns how to eat during the Appropriation Cycle, which is from 12 noon until 8 PM. Breakfast is taken care of, so basically we are talking about lunch and dinner. The goal is to eat in such a manner as to free energy from the digestive process, which in turn is used by the lymph system to regularly keep the body cleansed and free of waste. This will prevent toxins from ever again building up in the connective tissue. And that is precisely what is achieved by avoiding certain combinations of food, sometimes referred to as *proper food combining*.

Before continuing, I think it would be instructive to give you at least a brief bit of background on the concept of proper food combining. In 1985 the first **FIT FOR LIFE** book made quite a point of adhering to the principles of proper food combining. As the book's popularity grew, so did the rumblings from the people who never studied nutrition and the dietitians who are their allies. Proper food combining became ever so controversial. Not amongst the legions of people who were combining their foods properly and experiencing a dramatic improvement in their health, but from the professional negativists who "knew" proper food combining was worthless. How did they know this? Because they had not heard of it and it had never been part of their education.

In 1970, when I was 25 years old, I had never heard of it either. What I **had** heard of and was all too familiar with were Aspergum, Milk of Magnesia, Pepto-Bismol, and every other vile concoction that was poured down my throat to battle the excruciating pain in my stomach that had plagued me every single day of my life from the time I was three years old. For 22 years I never knew a single day's peace from these violent stomachaches. I had long given up any hope of ever being free of the pain. It had become a permanent part of my life. And all the doctors told me year after year was that I had a "sensitive stomach" and

I should just keep guzzling the nasty liquid chalk concoctions and learn to live with it.

Then in 1970, in a gift of grace, I was introduced to the work of an astounding human being named Herbert M. Shelton. No matter what flattering words I use to describe this extraordinary person, they will fall short of this colossus in the world of health. Surely the term *ahead of his time* was coined for just such a person as Herbert M. Shelton. Dr. Shelton lived from 1895 until 1985, and during that time, thanks to his towering intelligence and prodigious capacity for work, he earned half a dozen Ph.D.s and several lesser degrees in various areas of the healing arts. He authored over 40 books. For 31 years he wrote and published a monthly magazine. And for over 40 years he was the director of a Health School and Wellness Center in San Antonio, Texas, where he personally supervised and monitored the fasts and diets of over 50,000 people. Dr. Shelton is credited with being the driving force that took 150 years of research and writing on the subject of Natural Hygiene and unified it into a cohesive, scientific system of healing.

Some of his books are so innovative and ahead of their time that perhaps another 50 years or more will have to pass before the powers that be in the medical community come to realize just what a contribution he made to humankind. One of Dr. Shelton's primary areas of expertise was the workings of the human digestive tract, which he studied for over 60 years. No one before or since ever amassed such a vast body of knowledge on the subject. He knew, and proved beyond any possible doubt, the benefits to the body that resulted from the proper combination of foods.

In 1970 someone handed me a book by Dr. Shelton wherein he discussed the subject of proper food combining, and my life ever since has never been the same. **Thank God!** It was as though it was written specifically for my eyes. He explained that for some people who are particularly sensitive to ill-combined meals the result can be catastrophic. It doesn't affect everyone this way, but to those for whom it does, they could suffer with agonizing stomach and digestive disorders for years and never know what was beating them up. They merely resign themselves to swallowing repugnant concoctions to reduce the pain. Needless to say, he had my attention.

What he had to say about how one should combine foods, not only to relieve digestive disorders but also to conserve and boost energy seemed odd to me at the time because it was definitely contrary to the way that I ate. But I was willing to try anything under the sun that held even a **possibility** of removing the hot poker iron that was permanently lodged in my stomach.

No one can tell me that there's no such thing as miracles. In a matter of days I was free of pain and have not had a single stomachache since. The pain that had dogged me for over two decades was gone. It didn't go away gradually—it just stopped as though someone had turned off a big switch somewhere. For me proper food combining was a gift that was heaven-sent. That is why when I hear some medical doctor or poorly educated dietitian declare that proper food combining isn't scientific or some other inane criticism, I laugh out loud at them, as do hundreds of thousands of other people who know better. I figure their ancestors must be the people who "knew" Galileo was nuts and threw him into the dungeon for suggesting something as ridiculous as that it was the Earth circling the sun and not the other way around.

It's odd, but for some strange reason people tend to overcomplicate anything having to do with changes in their diet. I don't know why. I guess it's because people have somehow been convinced that figuring out a sensible, effective diet can't be simple. They're wrong. It can! I know that, depending on how technical the explanation is, proper food combining can become immensely confusing. I have heard some people describe it in ways that confuse me and I've been studying and teaching it for 35 years. Dozens of books on the subject have been written by authors all over the world, and I can tell you I'm glad they weren't the first introduction I had to it or I can't imagine that I ever would have taken to it the way I did.

I can't risk that happening to you. It's far too important and crucial to your success that you understand it and utilize it in your life. So I'm going to give you the most simple, straightforward, and uncomplicated version of proper food combining ever. The one most important underlying element to always bear in mind in overcoming Fibromyalgia, Lupus, Arthritis, or Chronic Fatigue Syndrome or any other malady of the body is that energy **must** be made available to the lymph system. Without energy, nothing will change, no progress will be made. The less work the digestive system has to perform; the more energy will be freed. It's as simple as that. And properly combining your foods definitely accomplishes that goal, as you will be able to verify for yourself after only a short while. Properly combining your foods will play a significant roll in overcoming Fibromyalgia, Lupus, Arthritis, and Chronic Fatigue Syndrome and preventing their return.

So here it is: Other than fruit, there are two types of food to eat—complex and simple. Complex foods are proteins (meat, chicken, fish, eggs, and dairy) and starches (bread, pasta, potatoes, and all grains). Simple foods are vegetables and salads. The complex foods (proteins and starches) require a great deal more digestive energy than do the simple foods (vegetables and salads). The idea is not to combine at the same meal two **different types** of complex foods but rather to have one type of complex food, **either** a protein **or** a starch, with vegetables and salad, which are the simple foods. That's it essentially.

It is best to not eat a protein together with a starch because they require different digestive juices. The digestive juice used to break down protein is acid. The digestive juice used to break down starch is alkaline. If you know anything about chemistry, you know that an acid and an alkaline mixed together neutralize each other. When that happens in the stomach, the digestive process is slowed and extended—exactly what you **don't** want. Proper food combining streamlines digestion—exactly what you **do** want.

In order to see to it that you are crystal clear on how to combine your meals properly, I'm going to give you some specific examples so you will clearly understand the process.

Let's say you want to have a steak. Since steak is a protein, you would not have starches such as potatoes or bread with it **at that meal**. Instead, you would have the steak with a vegetable or variety of vegetables prepared to your liking, along with a salad. You could even have an appetizer of shrimp cocktail, because it is also a protein. Same if you wanted broiled fish or grilled chicken or lamb chops. No starches with those proteins but rather vegetables and salad.

On the other hand, let's say that you are craving starches. You could have a nice bowl of pasta primavera, which means it has a lot of grilled vegetables mixed in with the pasta. You could also have garlic bread with it, because both pasta and bread are starches. And of course it should be accompanied by a salad.

If you are craving a baked potato, then have it with vegetables or stuffed mushrooms and a salad, which makes a delicious and satisfying meal. Also, when having a baked potato, if you want butter on it, by all means have it instead of margarine, which is nothing but plastic fat. Margarine is one of those horrific ploys that underhanded marketers use to trick you into thinking you're somehow doing something better for yourself than eating butter. At least butter is real. Margarine is disease waiting to happen. On those foods such as potato or other vegetables or on toast where you want butter, that's the way to go.

As you can see, there is no need to go hungry or be deprived of your favorites. You can eat and eat well. You just don't eat everything you like at every meal. You simply have proteins with vegetable and salad at one meal and starches with vegetable and salad at other meals. It may be different, but it's simple. The reason I differentiate salad from vegetables, even though salads **are** vegetables, is because when I talk about vegetables in terms of proper food combining I am referring to steamed, sautéed, baked, or otherwise cooked in some fashion. On the other hand when I talk about salads I am referring to vegetables that are uncooked and thereby totally living.

As important as it is to separate proteins and starches, it is equally important to have that salad with either. Remember, one of your goals is to make half of your diet living food. The salad is the living part, so don't pass on it in favor of the cooked foods. And please don't think that if you have a salad with lunch that you can't also have one with dinner. I'm astounded at how often I hear people say upon being asked if they want a salad, "No, thanks, I already had a salad today." **SO?!** I never hear people say upon being asked if they want a steak, "No, thanks, I already had meat today." In addition to the fruit you eat, salads are the living foods that your body is always craving. Don't look for reasons **not** to have them. Figure out how to have more of them.

Cravings being what they are, there will be occasions when one grabs hold of you and won't let go. That's life. You're going to want one of those traditional items that predominate the standard diet like a hamburger or pizza or cereal with milk, tuna fish or egg salad sandwich, ham and cheese, spaghetti and meatballs or a bagel with cream cheese. All are combinations of a protein and a starch. Everyone has these cravings. I know I do. You must be flexible with this approach to eating if it's going to work for you as a lifelong lifestyle. It's not what you do on occasion that will most impact your success; it's what you do consistently.

On those occasions when you strongly crave something, have it, enjoy it, and move on. It's not the end of the world. If you become fanatical, you're going to wind up frustrated and reverting back to the old way of eating. When you do have an ill-combined meal, there are some guidelines to follow to minimize their negative effect. First of all, if you should have an ill-combined meal for lunch, don't haul off and do it again at dinnertime. Make sure that the next meal is **not** one that overtaxes the digestive tract. In fact, to ensure the least negative effect from an ill-combined meal, the standing rule should be that at least a couple of days go by before doing it again. That way you're working in partnership with your body, and ill-combined meals once in a while simply will not be hurtful.

I've always loved eating sandwiches, but the traditional way always called for some kind of meat or cheese or both. So I've become fond of vegetable-based sandwiches. Sometimes I have a simple lettuce, tomato, and cucumber sandwich with mayo on whole wheat bread. Or I'll spread hummus on bread and add sliced-up artichoke hearts along with tomato or lettuce, and it's delicious. Or my favorite—avocado, lettuce, and tomato on whole wheat with a little mayo. You can become very creative, and that usually takes care of my desire for sandwiches. But sometime when nothing will do but one of those classically ill-combined sandwiches, I simply have it, enjoy it to the nth degree, and I don't need to do it again for a while. Depriving yourself of something you are truly craving is not healthy, so don't feel you have to do so.

I will tell you this, however. During the first six months when you are Mono-Dieting one week out of each month, that is the time to be the most disciplined of all. If you simply **must** have an ill-combined meal now and again, so be it. But try to your utmost to avoid them. That first six months is ever so crucial. Let's face it; Fibromyalgia, Lupus, Arthritis, and Chronic Fatigue Syndrome are not minor annoyances. They can, as you well know, take over your life and be terribly disruptive. They have so dumbfounded and bewildered members of the medical community that all they can tell you is there is no known cause, so take your drugs and live with it until a "cure" is found. I'm giving you a sensible, doable, tried, and proven means of overcoming these debilitating conditions, but you have to do your part, and that first six months requires your utmost committed effort.

I know full well that some people will say that having fruit for breakfast instead of the usual fare, and proper food combining are not scientific or some other such nonsense. I know that what I'm suggesting is the opposite of what most people do, and whenever you buck tradition and go against the grain by upsetting conventional thinking there will always be detractors who will do or say anything they have to in order to maintain the status quo. But their objections are based on long held, established dogma, **not** on personal experience. It's embarrassing for medical doctors to have someone outside the medical community come up with the answers that they were unable to provide.

If you jump from a tall building, whether you believe in gravity or not you are going to slam into the ground. Not believing in gravity or not accepting it as a reality will not protect you against the repercussions of denying its existence or pushing it beyond its limits. Ignoring, denying, or pretending that the principles governing the digestive tract are not real won't protect you against the inevitable results of their violation. The sooner you acknowledge, accept, and adhere to these principles the sooner you can start to be in charge of your well being.

What I am suggesting about fruit for breakfast and proper food combining proves itself. By doing it, you will feel better. If you feel better, will a doctor who never studied nutrition telling you it's not scientific make you stop doing what's working? I can remember several occasions in the past when I was on a TV or radio show being pitted against some medical doctor who knew practically nothing about nutrition. I would ask if s/he had ever tried for any length of time the suggestions that I was putting forth, and the patented, knee-jerk response was, "I don't have to; it's not based in science." In other words, "My mind is made up. Don't confuse me with the facts." As a point of interest Webster's dictionary defines science as "knowledge attained through study". Science is not the domain of the medical community; anyone can study and learn—that's science.

If you wanted to go on an extended sailing cruise to various ports of call, who would you want to take advice from about your trip—someone who has circumnavigated the planet on a sailboat? Or someone who had never even set foot on a sailing vessel of any kind?

I'm the one who has studied and taught this approach for 35 years and witnessed the success it can produce. All I'm asking from you is to try it and see for yourself. Besides, what alternatives are you being offered except for drugs and patience?

CHAPTER SEVEN

STEP THREE
TO RECOVERY

In the course of writing this book, the role and importance of two indispensable components have been
woven throughout. They are the underlying bedrock
foundation upon which any possible success in overcoming Fibromyalgia, Lupus, Arthritis, and Chronic
Fatigue Syndrome are based. And they are as insepa-
rable from each other as water is from the ocean. The
first is the vital importance of efficient and effective
digestion of food in the stomach. Precious few ailments of the human body cannot ultimately be traced
back to how well food was broken down and used by
the body. And the stomach is where it all starts.

The second is the incalculable role of living food, that is, foods with their enzymes intact. Enzymes are the living element in all life on the planet. Enzymes make food alive. Enzymes in food break down and digest the food when it enters the stomach. When living food is eaten, its enzymes are released, and digestion proceeds quickly, so the food spends the minimum amount of time in the stomach. When cooked food is eaten, meaning that its enzymes have been destroyed by the heat, the food sits around in the stomach waiting while the body exerts itself to produce the enzymes necessary to digest the food.

When cooked food predominates the diet, the repercussions of the body's being forced to produce the enzymes it needs on the spot go far beyond merely the unfortunate squandering of energy. As I stated earlier, the chain of events that unfolds as a result of digestion's being held up in the stomach can ultimately be linked to practically every malady of the human body.

Do you remember when I pointed out that food (other than fruit, of course) stays in the stomach for about three hours? That's in the best of circumstances. Depending upon what foods are eaten and in what combination, that time can double or even triple. When a protein and a starch are eaten at the same meal, in addition to the enzymes having been destroyed, the digestive juices that work in conjunction with enzymes are neutralized. It can get pretty foul in there. As the food sits around waiting for enzymes to be produced and sent to the stomach along with more digestive juices to replace the ones that were neutralized, the food starts to spoil. Don't forget, it's over 98 degrees in there, and hours are going by. Proteins will putrefy, and starches will ferment, contributing to the long list of digestive ailments for which billions upon billions of dollars are spent on drugs every year.

There is a perfect example I can use to clearly illustrate what I am talking about—one with which most everyone can relate. Although it's not a very pleasant subject of discussion, it is, nonetheless, an enormously instructive one.

One of those bodily functions that is reasonable to say most everyone has experienced at some point in time is the regurgitation of food—throwing up. Unpleasant though it may be to talk about, on the physiological level it speaks loudly to what can happen in the stomach when the digestive process is stalled for some reason.

Even though food needs to leave the stomach and enter the intestines as soon as possible, in approximately three hours, there are instances when people feel nauseous and throw up four, five, even six hours after eating. In some cases people will wake up in the morning and need to bolt out of bed and throw up food eaten seven or eight hours earlier. Something has to be seriously wrong for the body not to allow food to pass into the intestines and instead force it up and out of the body, and it's not a stomach virus, it's spoiled food. And what does vomit smell and taste like? You're probably "making a face" and cringing right now at the thought. **That's my point**. The body regurgitates food that is spoiled and foul, not fresh and wholesome.

Spoiled food cannot be built into healthy cell structure and support the body's needs, so it is expelled from the body, where it can do no harm. Precious energy is squandered on the entire process, energy that will not be available for the ever important process of healing. Even more frequently, food that has stayed in the stomach far longer than ideal is not thrown up but **is** passed into the intestines, where the body has to struggle to deal with it as best it can.

When food is efficiently and effectively digested in the stomach using a minimum of energy and then passed quickly into the intestines where the minimum amount of energy is used to extract what is needed, it bodes well for one's overall health. The energy not squandered unnecessarily on digestion in the stomach day after day for years on end translates into a considerable amount of energy that is available for use in removing toxins from the connective tissue and out of the body. What goes on in your stomach has a **direct** effect on overcoming Fibromyalgia, Lupus, Arthritis, and Chronic Fatigue Syndrome. Of that there is no doubt. **Anything** that can be done to facilitate digestion in the stomach **must** be undertaken and utilized. It would be foolish not to, wouldn't you think?

From the very beginning of my education in the 1970s, when I was first introduced to the work of Herbert M. Shelton, I became acutely aware of the enormous role that efficient digestion in the stomach plays in determining one's health. I had a desperate need at the time to find something that would ease me of my ills and lay the groundwork for a life free of pain and ill health.

The key was to find a way to streamline digestion as best I could. I knew that everything hinged on how quickly food left the stomach, and there were two primary reasons why food stayed in the stomach longer than necessary. The first was because of food spoiling due to ill-combined foods, causing digestive juices to neutralize. The second was due to the loss of naturally occurring digestive enzymes in food that were destroyed by the heat of cooking.

Fortunately, I learned about proper food combining, which, when practiced consistently, resolves the problem of food's spoiling in the stomach. From that time until today I have diligently followed the principle of proper food combining and have enjoyed the positive results of doing so. Out of an appreciation for the good that proper food combining has brought me, both in rescuing me from my stomach woes and increasing my overall level of energy, I decided to share the information with as many people as I could. Every **FIT FOR LIFE** book has at least some mention of the importance of properly combining foods.

It was the second factor that caused food to be held up in the stomach, the destruction of enzymes that pestered me. It was frustrating because I wanted to do what was best for my body, but once the enzymes are cooked away, that's it. The body has to take the time to produce its own; an energy squandering process. The only way to avoid the problem was to eat only living food. And although that would be a marvelously healthy way to eat, there was **no way** I was going to give up cooked food. Of course knowing that the more living food I ate and the less cooked food I ate the better off I'd be, I made sure that living food predominated my diet. At one point, as an experiment, I went on only living food for over a year. I felt beyond fantastic, but I missed cooked food so much that I was dreaming about it—while sleeping and while awake.

There was no other choice but to resign myself to the fact that cooked food had its price. Why do you think it is that the nutrient-supplement industry is a multibillion dollar one? The heat of cooking kills off so much of what we need in food that people try to make up for it by buying synthesized nutrients to make up for what is lost. Even if the manufactured nutrients were as good as what comes naturally in the food, which they aren't, not by a long shot, they still don't do anything to prevent the lag time in the stomach for food that has had its enzymes destroyed. So I simply ate more living food than cooked food and suggested that others do the same. Still, that nagging reality was always in the back of my mind, reminding me that every time I ate cooked food I was taxing my body's resources because of the longer length of time the food had to stay in the stomach. Yes, proper food combining helped, but there was no getting away from the fact that those enzymes were gone.

I used to actually fantasize about there being some kind of amazing discovery that was all natural and organic and would somehow prevent the enzymes in cooked food from being destroyed when heated. I also fantasized about winning the lottery.

My wishing, hoping, and fantasizing all came to a glorious end in 1995, when the universal powers that be finally answered my prayers. I could hardly believe it at the time, but I learned that there truly was a completely natural and organic product that actually did the work of the enzymes that are lost through cooking. I didn't want to allow myself to get too excited at first, just in case it was some hype or rip-off that is so common in the diet, health, and supplement industries. You

know, those commercials that come on showing someone wide-eyed and looking as if they're hyped up on
pure crystal caffeine and exclaiming that, "I lost 85
pounds and went down six dress sizes in just four
hours. Plus, I grew an extra arm!" Or, "You simply
attach these electrodes to your abdomen, and then sit
around watching TV and eating chocolate cheesecake.
When you stand up you'll have washboard abs."

I wanted to find out for myself everything I could
about this product. I had a trusted friend, who is as
much a stickler for purity as I, research it and see if it
was as good as advertised.

If you are at all familiar with my work over the
years, then you know that I'm not real big on pushing
scads of products. I could easily have my name or the
FIT FOR LIFE name on hundreds, literally hundreds,
of products due to the success of my books.

During the height of **FIT FOR LIFE**'s success,
when the book was not only on the *New York Times*
Best-seller List for two years but was also holding
down the coveted number-one position for ten straight
months, I was approached and asked to endorse more
nutritional supplement products than I could possibly
recall. In some instances I was told that I didn't have
to do anything but allow my name to be used, and I
could sit back and collect big, fat checks. I could have
put the money to good use, but I refused one and all. I

was much more interested in teaching people about the remarkable recuperative ability of the body and the proper way to eat in order to unleash its power.

I didn't want to push a lot of supplement products because, quite frankly, most of them are inferior. Did you know that research shows you have less of a chance of selecting nutritional products that are both non-toxic and effective, than ones that are? That means you have to be ever diligent to avoid selecting nutritional products that are either toxic or don't work.

Due to my difficulties with Agent Orange poisoning I have to be ultra careful about what I put into my body. Ingesting toxic substances in my case could be life-threatening. So **no way** would I ever recommend a nutritional product to someone that I myself would not use. I am one of those people who is firmly convinced that we are here to help others, not take advantage of them.

I don't want to imply that there are no good nutritional products to be had; that would be ridiculous. After all, excellent products do exist. I don't want to be so rigid and closed-off to nutritional products that I miss out on something that could actually help me. Sometimes something comes along that is of such immense worth and value that it would be foolish not to make use of it. You have likely heard the old adage, "If something seems to be too good to be true, it probably is." The operative word in that sentence is "probably". In most cases that which appears to be too good to be true really is, but there are also those rare occasions when something shows up that truly is every bit as good as the buildup. I am ever so pleased to tell you about one of those.

The product to which I am referring is called *Live Plant Digestive Enzymes*. The result of my friend conducting exhaustive research revealed that thanks to some impressive headway being made in the task of producing nutritional products, a product of unsurpassed purity and effectiveness had been developed that overcame the problem of enzymes in cooked food being destroyed by heat.

Research on enzyme nutrition has been ongoing for over half a century. The person most credited with unlocking the mystery of enzymes is Dr. Edward Howell, who lived from 1898 to 1991 and is recognized as the expert's expert when it comes to understanding enzymes. His book, *Enzyme Nutrition*, in 1985 is considered to be the "Bible" on the subject. It is a fascinating book that explains everything you would ever want to know about enzymes.

Live Plant Digestive Enzymes come in very small capsules that are to be taken immediately before eating anything cooked. They are specifically formulated to fulfill the role of the food enzymes destroyed in the cooking process. So, instead of food's sitting around in the stomach, waiting while the body scrambles to produce the enzymes needed for digestion and depleting its own limited resources, the digestive enzymes go straight to work on the food as soon as it enters the stomach. There is no lag time, so the food spends the least amount of time in the stomach as possible. All the problems associated with delayed digestion and the unnecessary squandering of energy are avoided. This, of course, has the much desired effect of freeing energy for use by the lymph system to work on cleansing. Plus, many of the problems of indigestion that are the result of digestion's being held up are prevented.

I set about to locate the absolute finest and purest Live Plant Digestive Enzymes available anywhere on the planet. Thanks in part to my years of association with some of the top people in the health and fitness world, I was successful in my efforts. It turns out that the highest-quality Digestive Enzymes are produced in Japan. After reading about the research, development, experimentation, and studies done on the university level and the experiences of numerous people who used Live Plant Digestive Enzymes, I was satisfied that this was the genuine article.

I started using Live Plant Digestive Enzymes in mid-1995, and the difference in the way it made, and continues to make me feel after eating cooked food, is like the proverbial night and day. It really has to be experienced to be fully appreciated. I have heard comments from people who started using Digestive Enzymes that you would surely think were exaggerations. The words, "Miracle" or "Godsend" became almost commonplace. One person told me that after decades of feeling bloated, gassy, and heavy after every meal, she had given up the idea of feeling any other way. From the very first meal when she started using Digestive Enzymes she was transformed as though by magic. She didn't realize that she could actually feel light after a meal.

Another person told me that Digestive Enzymes brought the joy back to eating. For years he would rarely eat one of his favorite foods, pizza, because of how he felt after doing so. He said that the first time he ate pizza after taking the Digestive Enzymes first, he sat, antacids in hand, waiting for the inevitable cramps and pain that **always** followed. When they didn't occur he felt as though he had discovered the Holy Grail.

Yet another person told me that whenever she ate she didn't even wait for the customary discomfort. She would simply finish her meal and swallow her antacids. Upon first learning about Digestive Enzymes she was actually scared not to take the antacids after eating, because she "knew" how painful and uncomfortable it would be for her. When the usual discomfort failed to materialize, it was for her a miracle.

Many others commented on the various improvements and well-being they experienced as a result of food's being digested in the stomach quickly without it's having to sit around waiting for the body to replace the enzymes destroyed by cooking.

When you hear stories like this over and over from people of all different walks of life, it becomes apparent that this is one of those rare instances when a product actually delivers on its promises.

There are estimates that declare that 60% of those diagnosed with Fibromyalgia also have chronic digestive disorders.[40] The people who "don't know" will tell you that no one knows why Fibromyalgia, Lupus, and Chronic Fatigue Syndrome patients have such a high incidence of digestive disorders. In actuality, there is a reasonable and logical reason why the number is so high. Frankly, as disturbing as the number is, I was surprised that it wasn't even higher. After all, Fibromyalgia, Lupus, Arthritis, and Chronic Fatigue Syndrome are the result of a prolonged and neglected buildup of toxins. We know that two of the highest priorities of the body in terms of where to allocate available energy are the digestion of food and the cleansing of toxins so that they don't imperil health. These two priorities are always vying for whatever energy is available.

Since Fibromyalgia, Lupus, Arthritis, and Chronic Fatigue Syndrome are the **end** result of the prolonged buildup of toxins, which means that the body's health is in jeopardy, every effort will be made to find the energy necessary to lower the level of toxins. It stands to reason that if the body determines that the need to remove toxins has reached the urgency level, as is the case with Fibromyalgia, Lupus, Arthritis, and Chronic Fatigue Syndrome, the function of the body that uses the greatest amount of energy, digestion, will have to relinquish some of its allotment. The battle for energy rages and digestion suffers, resulting in chronic digestive disorders.

The fact that there is something that dramatically diminishes the energy requirement for digestion translates into a tremendous boon for the cleansing and healing efforts of the body. That is what Live Plant Digestive Enzymes succeed in doing. The process that devours most of the energy is when cooked food first enters the stomach and the realization hits that the enzymes needed to digest it are not there. The effort that the body **must** make to somehow produce the necessary enzymes and speed them to the stomach is what gobbles up so much energy. By taking Digestive Enzymes immediately before eating cooked food, the entire problem is eliminated, because the enzymes are already in the stomach waiting for the food. Digestion proceeds in a smooth, efficient, and timely fashion. Live Plant Digestive Enzymes are nothing short of a gift from on high in terms of what those suffering from

Fibromyalgia, Lupus, Arthritis, and Chronic Fatigue Syndrome are trying to accomplish.

Two factors of great importance must be considered when choosing Digestive Enzymes: purity and potency. The Digestive Enzymes that I sought out, researched, and decided to use exclusively and will be advising you to use as well are, I can assure you, the absolute finest available in the world. I will acknowledge that Live Plant Digestive Enzymes of **equal** purity and potency may exist, but there are none that are superior.

Since I am recommending that you start using Digestive Enzymes whenever eating cooked food, I want to very briefly tell you of their purity and potency so you can feel confident and assured that they will do only good in your body. There are two types of Digestive Enzymes: pharmaceutical and commercial. The ones I use and recommend are, of course, pharmaceutical-grade. They are harvested from 100% organically grown plants (aspergillus) and formulated in the most pristine conditions in a laboratory setting. No heat, solvents, or chemicals of any kind are used. There are no additives or anything artificial used in any stage of their growing, harvesting, or formulation. Even the tiny capsules they come in are made from vegetable cellulose, not gelatin from cow or horse hooves, so there is no chance of any contamination with *e.coli*, salmonella, listeria, mad cow, etc.

As regards potency, you may presently be aware of Digestive Enzymes that are on the market. There is no comparison to Live Plant Digestive Enzymes. Commercially made enzymes produced from papaya or pineapple fall far short of pharmaceutical-grade enzymes. First of all, they are primarily designed to help in digesting protein and only minimally help with fat and starches. Live Plant Digestive Enzymes digest all three. Also, store-bought Digestive Enzymes are sold by weight in milligrams, so you don't actually know what you're getting. They can have fillers, additives, cornstarch, or any number of other ingredients taking up space in the capsules. The actual amount of enzyme could be miniscule, which is generally the case. Live Plant Digestive Enzymes are sold by what is referred to as *units of activity*. No fillers, no additives: nothing but pure enzyme, with a potency far, far in excess of commercial enzymes sold off the shelf in health food stores, drugstore chains, or on infomercials. What you are getting is all enzyme and absolutely nothing else, which is why the capsules are so small.

In my opinion the discovery of Live Plant Digestive Enzymes is the single greatest achievement in the area of diet and health since we humans started eating cooked food. From that day in 1995 when I first discovered that these Digestive Enzymes were available, until today, I have not had a single cooked meal in which I did not take my Digestive Enzymes. Not **one**. And I cannot imagine myself ever doing differently. I would rather not eat at all than eat cooked food without them. I take them with me when I travel, when I eat out in restaurants, or when invited to friends' homes for dinner. And I am strongly urging you to do the same.

I know that I am asking you to go to the expense of purchasing them, but fortunately they are quite inexpensive, especially when compared to drugs to combat the problems that Digestive Enzymes prevent. These drugs are three, sometimes four times the cost, and not only do they not address the cause of the problem but they actually **add** toxins to the body. When measured against the benefits that Live Plant Digestive Enzymes produce, the cost is practically incidental. Plus, I have made special arrangements so that anyone ordering Digestive Enzymes as a result of reading this book will receive a discount on their purchase.

To obtain your Live Plant Digestive Enzymes, call toll free: 877-335-1509 or go to our website: www.fitforlifetime.com.

If you will commit to Mono-Dieting in the manner in which I have suggested, eating fruit till noon, combining your foods as I have recommended when not Mono-Dieting, and using Live Plant Digestive Enzymes whenever eating cooked food, I can tell you that your health and your life will be transformed. Other people in your situation have made significant headway in dealing with Fibromyalgia, Lupus, Arthritis, and Chronic Fatigue Syndrome by incorporating this approach to eating into their lifestyle, and no good reason on Earth exists why you cannot join their ranks.

Think of what your alternative is: allowing your condition to worsen unabated with no letup in sight. As the medical community shrugs its collective shoulders declaring that "no one knows" the cause of Fibromyalgia, Lupus, Arthritis, and Chronic Fatigue Syndrome, the **entire** thrust in dealing with them is to throw drugs at the problem. Go on the internet or to the library and look up your specific condition and see for yourself. **Everything** revolves around drugs to manage, cope with, or in some way learn how to live with pain. Every supposed advance made is associated with some new drug that may diminish the pain. Not a single, solitary word is **ever** uttered about the possibility of actually understanding what causes these devastating illnesses and overcoming or preventing them. As far as the medical community and the pharmaceutical industry are concerned it's business as usual.

As a perfect example of what I am talking about, a nationwide survey commissioned by the Arthritis Foundation shows that 70 percent of adults in the United States with Rheumatoid Arthritis still experience joint pain, stiffness and fatigue on a daily basis. In response to this, Dr. John H. Klippel, president and CEO of the Arthritis Foundation stated that, "This survey brings to light the need for aggressive research to improve the treatment of Rheumatoid Arthritis. It is a clear indication that we still have a great deal of work to do to improve quality of life for people with Rheumatoid Arthritis when more than two-thirds of the people surveyed experience symptoms that limit their ability to perform daily activities, in spite of taking their medication."[41]

You See? Every word spoken by this gentleman has to do with "treatment" and the need for new drugs to "improve quality of life" because they are still suffering greatly "in spite of taking their medication." There isn't even a hint of an inference to the possibility of actually rescuing these people from the disease itself.

At least what I am offering you within these pages gives you some hope of understanding why you have the symptoms you do and a strategy for removing them. And it's not with some goofy, non-sensible approach that defies reason, is difficult to undertake, and has negative side effects. Besides, what harm could there possibly be in improving the quality of your diet? Drugs have negative side effects that can severely harm you or kill you, improving your diet has no such side effects. Plus, as you can see from Dr. Klippel's statement, the drugs aren't even helping in

70% of the cases. It's not as though I just made this stuff up out of the blue and am guessing that it **might** help, it has a track record of helping people and not hurting anyone. Let's see if we can add you to that list.

Before leaving the subject of enzymes I wish to invite you to read Appendix I in the back of the book (page 307) where you will learn some fascinating and valuable information about enzymes and the vital and essential role they play in every aspect of your life. You will also learn about two sensational new, natural enzyme products recently made available that actually reduces inflammation in the body without all the negative side effects commonly associated with anti-inflammatory drugs.

CHAPTER EIGHT

THIS, THAT,
AND THE OTHER

I wish to share with you a few items of importance that will support your effort in all of this—some helpful hints that will add to your success in reaching your goal of reducing or removing pain from your life.

One. There is a good reason why anyone who knows anything about diet and health, and even those who don't, try to discourage the eating of fried foods. They are extremely counterproductive to a healthy life. Fried foods supply nothing of worth to the body but plenty that is harmful, and they overwork and pollute the digestive tract. Foods soaked in oils at a high temperature wreak havoc in the body. The goal should be to see what can be done to give the digestive system less work, not more. Foods like fried chicken or fish, French fries, onion rings, chips, and doughnuts are all foods that sabotage your success. I'm not suggesting that you never have them, only that you be aware of their harmfulness and minimize their consumption. Especially during the first six months when it is so critical to support your body's efforts in any way you can.

Two. In Step Two to Recovery I discussed the most perfect and beneficial food one can eat. The one, when correctly eaten, which will help you overcome Fibromyalgia, Lupus, Arthritis, and Chronic Fatigue Syndrome more than any other: fruit. Now I need to tell you about the food that is the exact polar opposite of fruit, the one that is, in my opinion, the worst, and most harmful food in the human diet. The one that contributes to ill health more than any other food: dairy products.

If you are not one of those people fortunate enough to have learned the truth about this agent of ill health and disease, you may be shocked or even think that I have a screw loose somewhere at what I am saying. People only continue to consume dairy products in the massive amounts that they do because they are the victims of one of the most successful and cruel cashectomies ever devised in all the history of commerce. A cashectomy is the process of convincing you to hand over hefty fistfuls of your hard-earned cash for a product or service you are convinced will in some way improve your life and well-being and receiving instead something that hurts you, makes you sick, or kills you. You may not be aware of it, but cashectomies are being performed on you every single day: baby formulas, breakfast cereals, margarine, pasteurized orange juice sold as "all natural," Lunchables, most drugs. The list goes on and on. And one of the most successful and long-running ones is dairy products.

Whatever you have heard about the "benefits" of dairy products is a big, fat lie. It's not the result of a mistake in understanding or the result of all the evidence not being in yet, it's the result of a deliberate, unabashed, bold-faced lie devised to make billions of dollars. One of the most despised figures in all of history once said, "If you tell a lie big enough, loud enough, long enough, and often enough, the people will believe it." That was Adolf Hitler, and it describes perfectly the con job that has been foisted onto an innocent and trusting public regarding dairy products. If people knew the real truth, they would be lined up to sue the dairy industry the same way they are to sue the tobacco industry.

I really have to start learning how to express myself without beating around the bush and stop being evasive and wishy-washy when it comes to declaring my true feelings on subjects like this.

In some of my past books I went into the subject of dairy products in great detail, bringing to bear the titanic body of evidence proving my point. I discussed not only the data that backed up and proved my position but also the politics and behind-the-scenes shenanigans associated with tricking you into believing that dairy products are, of all things, good for you. I'm not going to do that again here. Instead I'm merely going to give you a little common sense evidence for you to contemplate. Anyone can hire an "expert" to say anything true **or** false about a given product, so long as the price is right. But common sense cannot be bartered. Common sense is the great enemy of the cashectomists plying their trade in the dairy industry.

God's exquisite and supremely intelligent plan for newborn mammals (humans included) is a milk that is the perfect **first** food. Every species of mammal has its own unique and perfect milk for its young. Elephants and mice are both mammals, and the way the Grand Creator of all and everything worked it out, one milk is unique and perfect for building a huge body with massive bones while the other is unique and perfect for building a small body with more delicate bones. Giraffe milk is unique and perfect for baby giraffes. Water buffalo milk is unique and perfect for baby water buffalos. Whale milk is unique and perfect for baby whales. Cow milk is unique and perfect for baby cows. And human milk is unique and perfect for baby humans. And as is with Nature's plan with hundreds upon hundreds of different mammal species, **ALL** stop consuming milk once they are weaned, never to drink milk again. Not the milk of their own species or of any other species.

The one and only exception to this grand plan, the one species of mammal to go against nature and continue drinking milk, even after being weaned, is human. As wrong as that is, humans don't even drink the milk of their own species but a milk from a species with which they have nothing in common insofar as the size, shape, and needs of each.

A baby cow weighs about 90 pounds at birth and will attain the weight of between one and two thousand pounds in **only two years**. A baby human weighs about five to ten pounds at birth and will reach a weight of between one and two hundred pounds in **18 years**. The milk needed by these two different species is completely different. Calves, once weaned, will not drink milk, even when offered milk from their own mother. **That's because milk is the food intended for babies, not adults**.

Don't think for a moment that this obvious, common sense argument wasn't a huge obstacle for the dairy cashectomists to overcome. They had to come up with something to persuade people to actually go against their true nature and God's grand plan. It wasn't easy, but when billions of dollars are at stake some of the most deviously creative minds can be hired and brought to bear. An ingenious scheme was hit upon that unfortunately was swallowed hook, line, and milk bucket.

What better way to get people to consume a product than to convince them that without it they will suffer terribly from a painful and debilitating disease: osteoporosis. Women in particular have been preyed upon by this scheme by holding the threat of osteoporosis over their head like an executioner's axe.

Calcium is the number-one mineral, by quantity, needed by the human body. Cow's milk contains a rich source of calcium in order to build the comparatively massive bones it needs. It was a simple leap to tell folks that cow's milk was not only a good source of calcium **for humans** but also that without it their bones would become as brittle as kindling.

Never mind that the calcium in cow's milk is uniquely structured for cows and can't be used by humans. Never mind that the protein component in milk, casein, is the base for one of the strongest wood glues in existence and there's 300 times more casein in cow's milk than in human milk. Never mind that dairy products are high in fat and cholesterol and devoid of fiber, the exact opposite combination of what is recommended by every health authority the world over. Never mind that Americans consume an astounding 125 **billion** pounds of dairy products a year and still have one of the highest incidences of osteoporosis in the world. All of these facts took a backseat to profits.

The most reprehensible aspect of the dairy cashectomy is the tactic of holding the specter of osteoporosis over the heads of people when enough data exists to bury a herd of cows that proves undeniably that dairy products **contribute** to osteoporosis. Not that it's the only cause, but dairy products contribute very significantly to osteoporosis. And yet it is marketed as a means of helping **prevent** the disease. Now that is a first-rate cashectomy that must have professional cashectomists whoopin' and hollerin' and high-fivein' one another all over the world.

The four countries of the world that consume the greatest number of dairy products per capita are the United States, Great Britain, Sweden, and Finland.[42] The four countries of the world that suffer the highest incidence of osteoporosis are, well, what do you know, the United States, Great Britain, Sweden, and Finland.[43] Now you don't think that just happens to be an ironic coincidence, do you?

The countries of the world that consume the least dairy products are the African and Asian countries,[44] and wouldn't you know it, they also happen to be the countries with the least incidence of osteoporosis.[45] Gee, another astounding coincidence.

China is the most heavily populated country on Earth, with 1.3 billion people. That's a billion people more than the entire population of the United States. The Chinese people don't like dairy products. They think dairy smells and tastes funny, so they leave it alone. Osteoporosis is so uncommon in China that there's no word for it in their language![46]

These facts I am relating to you are undeniable and unassailable truths. They cannot be covered up, and they cannot be explained away by the dairy industry's hired apologists. And an army of medical doctors who have never studied nutrition, dietitians who are in bed with the dairy industry, and a thousand famous celebrities with a milk mustache are not going to alter that fact one bit.

I have to share a story with you that I will never forget. Sometime in the late 1980s I received a letter from a woman who wrote that the letter I was reading was the first letter she had written in nearly ten years. She said that she had Arthritis so bad in her hands that she couldn't hold a pen to write. After reading **FIT FOR LIFE** she made only two changes. She ate only fruit in the morning instead of the usual oatmeal and toast, and she cut out **all** dairy products. It only took a few short months and she was able to hold a pen and wanted me to be the first person she wrote.

I'm not suggesting that you give up all dairy products. What I'm telling you comes under the category of "know thy enemy." Dairy products place an extremely heavy burden on the digestive process, the exact opposite of what you want, so cut back. That's all I'm suggesting.

If you do have a concern about Calcium, do what the Chinese people do. They get all the Calcium they need from the plant kingdom. Every food that grows from the ground has some calcium in it, so eat a well-rounded diet that includes living food, and you will get all the Calcium you need. One of the benefits of eating a diet that is half living food and half cooked food is that you will ingest all of the vitamins and minerals your body needs, including calcium.

If you want to take a calcium supplement, just "to be sure," you can use a high-quality coral Calcium, which is a totally naturally occurring Calcium that is utilized perfectly by the body without any of the problems associated with dairy products or with Calcium from crushed rocks or seashells. Check the contact page at the end of the book, and I will tell you how to get information on the coral Calcium I use and recommend to my readers, or you may call toll-free 877-335-1509 or go to our website: www.fitforlifetime.com. I also invite you to read Appendix II (page 327) for a more detailed discussion of the subject of Coral Calcium.

One last thought to contemplate about dairy products and Calcium: Since cows never drink milk after being weaned at about six months old, where do they get all that perfect Calcium? **From plants!** The same as elephants, and look at their bones.

Three. If you are presently smoking cigarettes you certainly don't need me to tell you to stop. I'm sure you're already aware of all the dangers associated with smoking and in all likelihood would like to stop for those reasons. So I'm not going to go into a full-court press in an attempt to persuade you to stop. But I do have to bring up the subject briefly.

There's no easy or diplomatic way to bring this up, so I'm just going to come out with it. Your challenge to overcome Fibromyalgia, Lupus, Arthritis, and Chronic Fatigue Syndrome is increased tenfold, if not more, if you are smoking. It's probably not something you want to hear, but I wouldn't want you to think that your slow progress was due to the principles I've shared with you not working as well as I have stated they would.

Let me explain why smoking puts the brakes on success as much as it does, because it's probably something you have not heard before. Oxygenated blood must reach and nourish every last cell on the inside of your body. If not, those cells not regularly nourished with oxygenated blood will die. That is why there are over **90,000 miles** of blood vessels in your body. If blood flow is restricted, for whatever reason, bad things start to happen. It is no surprise that cardiovascular disease (heart attacks, arterioschlerosis, atheroschlerosis, strokes) is the greatest killer of all time, taking approximately a million lives a year in the United States alone. That is more than all other causes of death by disease **combined**. That's over 2,700 people dying every single day.

With **every** drag of smoke that is inhaled, all 90,000 miles of blood vessels simultaneously constrict. Every one! When blood vessels constrict, blood flow is restricted. That means every last activity of the body is impeded. Every organ is prevented from operating at full capacity. The heart, lungs, liver, kidneys, spleen— everything is prevented from performing its part in keeping the living body alive. Digestion is slowed, as is the work of the lymph system, and those are the two functions of the body that **must** be completely unfettered to have any hope of overcoming Fibromyalgia, Lupus, Arthritis, and Chronic Fatigue Syndrome.

A recent study has revealed that Smoking **greatly** increases the risk of Rheumatoid Arthritis among people with a genetic predisposition for the disease.[47] No matter what your health goals, smoking can only hurt your chances of success.

The good news I can give you if you are smoking and you want to commit yourself to overcoming

Fibromyalgia, Lupus, Arthritis, and Chronic Fatigue Syndrome with the principles you have learned here is the fact that you weren't born a smoker. Air is the number-one prerequisite for life to continue. About six minutes without air, and the body dies. The body itself will go to great lengths to protect the lungs and keep them functioning as effectively as possible. When you start to eat more living food by Mono-Dieting, eating fruit correctly and in the morning hours, properly combining proteins and starches, and using Live Plant Digestive Enzymes when eating cooked food, the body starts to heal itself with the newfound energy that this way of eating produces. You will automatically have fewer cravings for cigarettes.

No less than a dozen people have written to tell me that without doing anything more than following the recommendations you have learned in this book, they gradually smoked less and less until finally quitting altogether. In one instance a woman told me she had smoked two packs a day for **27 years** before quitting. As she became more and more healthy, cigarettes became increasingly distasteful to her. Finally she quit because she couldn't stand the taste. Your body is your greatest ally and will work in your behalf in a never ending quest to optimize health. If you will do your part by properly feeding your body, your body will most assuredly do its part.

Four. In talking about the extreme importance of oxygenated blood's reaching all the cells of the body,

I must make a quick point about exercise. You don't have to become a world-class athlete in order to satisfy the body's need for exercise, but some minimal amount of physical activity is essential. The greatest eating plan on Earth will accomplish only so much without the benefit of some regular exercise.

In one alarming study released by the government, it was revealed that 55% of adults don't get the minimum amount of exercise of 30 minutes a day at least four times a week.[48] That's one out of every two adults that are not doing the barest minimum. And that's counting activities such as gardening, housework, waiting tables, throwing a Frisbee, mowing the lawn, and washing the car as exercise. That is sorrowful, to say the least.

You might be surprised to learn how little exercise is actually needed in order to meet the body's needs. If you are already doing something regularly such as walking, jogging, biking, swimming, rebounding, tennis, or any combination of different exercises, that's fine. It's all you need. But if you are doing **nothing**, your chances of success of overcoming Fibromyalgia, Lupus, Arthritis, and Chronic Fatigue Syndrome will be lessened even if you follow the dietary guidelines explicitly.

The human body is built for movement, so muscles must be used, or else they deteriorate. If you were to put one of your arms in a sling and not use it for several months, when you took the sling off you would find that the muscles had atrophied from nonuse and your arm had withered. Guess what? The heart is the strongest muscle in the human body, and it needs regular exercise.

The one vigorous, physical activity that can bring you and your heart all the benefits produced by exercise can be done practically anywhere at anytime by nearly anyone, regardless of physical condition. It doesn't require elaborate facilities or equipment and is convenient and easy. I'm referring to walking. Walking produces results in short-term training and in long-term health benefits equal to any other aerobic exercise—including jogging.[49]

Over the last 10 years or so, an immense amount of data has come forth from the scientific community showing that even the most moderate, unstructured walking program will reap significant benefits. Not only are low levels of activity beneficial but the benefits are cumulative. In other words, if you took three ten-minute, brisk walks during the course of the day, the benefits would be the same as if you took one thirty-minute walk.

I want to tell you of another extremely important reason why a minimum amount of exercise is necessary. Unlike the cardiovascular system, which has the heart pumping blood throughout the body, the lymph system has no such pump; it is dependant upon physical activity in order to keep lymph flowing through the body.

As you have learned throughout this book, the way to overcome Fibromyalgia, Lupus, Arthritis, and Chronic Fatigue Syndrome depends upon two crucial factors. First, the digestive process must be streamlined so as not to squander precious energy that can be used in healing. Second, the lymph system must function at its highest efficiency so it can remove toxins from the connective tissue and the body. The formula is simple: the less physical activity, the less the lymph system will be able to accomplish. The more physical activity, the better the lymph system will function. This is no small matter. Some minimum amount of physical activity is a must.

What I suggest is that you make the time to take a brisk 20-to-30 minute walk every day or at the very **least** every other day. This will stimulate and benefit both the heart and the lymph system. Or, if you prefer, you can have a rebounder (mini-trampoline) in your home and gently bounce up and down on it for short periods of time a few times during the day, and that will also reap enormous rewards. I have been rebounding daily for over 20 years, because not only is it a great aerobic exercise but it also stimulates and pumps the lymph system.

Considering its convenience and the benefits it reaps, rebounding has to be one of the most worthwhile physical activities in existence. To learn more about obtaining the REBOUND*AIR* Rebounder I use you may call toll-free 877-335-1509 or go to our website: www.fitforlifetime.com.

As you can see, there are easy and convenient ways of fulfilling your body's need for exercise. Nothing is easier or comes more naturally than walking. Make the effort; do it to help your body in its efforts to help you feel better. Don't put it off—start **today**. It's that important.

Five. The challenge of reducing the incidence of pain in America isn't confined only to understanding and overcoming Fibromyalgia, Lupus, Arthritis, and Chronic Fatigue Syndrome. Although they do account for a very significant amount of the pain and discomfort people must deal with on a regular basis, there are other causes as well. I wish to touch on two of those briefly because they are two of the most common of all complaints: headaches and lower back pain.

Headaches are the number one cause of pain in the U.S. Since the point of view put forth in this book is that of the field of Natural Hygiene, it is from that perspective the cause and prevention of headaches are discussed. The most prominent types of headaches are cluster, congestive, migraine, tension, throbbing, and toxic. But determining the different types of headaches is secondary to the fact that the causes are essentially the same.

In the midst of a particularly brutal headache it can feel like your entire brain is pounding and in pain. Interestingly, however, the brain does not experience pain. A headache is pain that occurs only in the scalp **outside** of the cranium (the part of the skull that encases and protects the brain). Most headaches involve pulsating pain, that is, throbbing. This is an indication that the periodic surges of blood with each heartbeat aggravate and intensify the pain.

The actual mechanical cause of a headache is the constriction or partial closure of blood vessels leading to the brain. This tightening of the blood vessels restricts blood flow into the cranium causing the retention of blood in the blood vessels around the cranium. This can result in pressure that makes it seem like something is going to explode. It is this increased blood pressure around the cranium that is the source of headache pain.

Why would the intelligent body do this to itself? Why would it so constrict blood vessels as to restrict blood flow to the brain? The answer lies in the fact that the brain is the most vital organ of the entire body, and therefore is the most protected organ of the body. As strange as it might sound, a headache is a defensive,

protective measure used by the intelligent body to protect the brain from harm. And what specifically is the
body trying to protect the brain against? The very
same thing that inflames connective tissue: toxins. It is
therefore not surprising that one of the symptoms of
those with connective tissue disorders (Fibromyalgia,
Lupus, and Arthritis) is headaches.

As is the case with Fibromyalgia, Lupus, Arthritis,
and Chronic Fatigue Syndrome, a headache is merely
the symptom of an underlying cause, that cause being
toxins that could harm the brain. Caffeine, nicotine,
alcohol, soft drinks, food additives, refined sugar,
chemicals, pesticides, prescribed and over-the-counter
drugs, and the biggest culprit of all, the dietary intake
of refined and processed cooked foods, all contribute
to the level of toxins in the body that lead to pain. A
headache is the brain protecting itself from these toxic
substances that ultimately wind up in the blood.

I told you earlier of the tremendous amount of
feedback I have received in the form of over a half
million letters from people who have read my books.
In literally thousands of those letters people spoke of
how delighted they were that they no longer had the
headaches that used to be so commonplace. Many told
me that even the migraines they used to have, the most
painful and unbearable of all headaches, have either
greatly diminished or stopped altogether. One woman
told me that she had suffered with migraines almost

daily for 17 years! Having experienced migraines earlier in my life I could hardly believe that she endured
them for that long. She wrote me a very long, hand-
written letter expressing her overwhelming joy at not
having a single migraine headache for weeks on end
after closely following the approach to eating you
have read about here.

There are several reasons why someone may experience, ongoing lower back pain, other than the pain
that might occur from some kind of injury. The pain
could be associated with the connective tissue inside
of a muscle (Fibromyalgia), or in the tendons, ligaments, or supportive connective tissue (Lupus), or in
one of the many joints of the lower back, or pelvis, or
where the two are joined together (Arthritis).
Everything you have learned about cleansing and healing the connective tissue in this book would certainly
address these causes.

There is yet another cause for sharp and piercing
lower back pain with which I am all too familiar: a
pinched nerve. Your spinal cord is a glistening white
bundle of nerves, which runs from your brain down a
canal in your *spinal column*, or backbone, which is
made up of 31 small interlocking, movable bones
called *vertebrae*. There is a small opening between
each vertebra through which nerves branch off and
travel to different parts of the body. A vertebra can lose
its proper position and become misaligned with the

vertebrae above and below it, and clamp down on, or pinch, a nerve and cause considerable pain. The actual amount of movement necessary for a vertebra to move and pinch a nerve is extremely small. If you have never experienced the knife-like, stabbing pain that a pinched nerve can cause, I say thank goodness for you, and I hope it is something you never do experience.

I wish I could tell you that I have no first hand knowledge of pain from a pinched nerve, but, well, I do. I shared with you earlier the circumstances surrounding my experience with Agent Orange-induced peripheral neuropathy. There are striking similarities between peripheral neuropathy and amyotrophic lateral sclerosis (ALS) or what is commonly referred to as Lou Gehrig's Disease. With Lou Gehrig's, muscles all deteriorate simultaneously. With peripheral neuropathy it is more haphazard; some muscles will atrophy and disappear while muscles right next to them are unaffected. This has set up an interesting dynamic in my body in that muscles that are intact pull my spine out of alignment because the muscles that would offset this are gone. The result is a vertebra moving ever so slightly and pinching a nerve.

Ordinarily a simple chiropractic adjustment would realign the vertebra, releasing the nerve. And although I received these adjustments on a regular basis, with good results, the relief was only temporary because of my extraordinary circumstances with peripheral neuropathy.

There was a period of about four years where my lower back hurt so bad that I was actually disappointed to wake up in the morning. It's the kind of pain that takes over your life; you can't think of anything else.

Then, in what can only be described as an answer to prayer, I was introduced to an apparatus called an Inversion Table.

This is a lightweight but sturdy apparatus on which you lie flat on your back with your ankles held in place. By moving your arms up or down you can tilt your body anywhere from slightly past horizontal to fully upside down. Spending even a very short time upside down has some extremely beneficial effects,

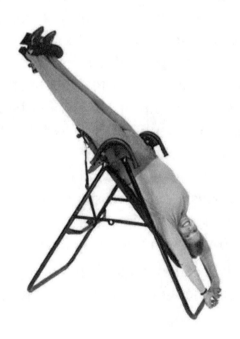

not the least of which is to gently stretch the spine which in turn separates and aligns the vertebrae so as to not clamp down on nerves!

When I first heard about the particular benefit of pinched nerves being released I quickly became a man on a mission. I did not allow another moment to pass before finding out where I could obtain an Inversion Table even if there was only a remote chance at best that I could find some relief for my back. I located one 60 miles from where I live and jumped into my car and drove like a madman to go pick it up. How I managed to go and return without receiving a speeding ticket I'll never know because I was haulin' the entire trip up and back.

I set the table up and climbed on. At first it was a bit disconcerting because I was not accustomed to having so much blood in my head and quite frankly I could only remain upside down for 20 or 30 seconds without feeling like blood was going to start shooting out my ears. But I took it slowly and before long I could go upside down for as long as I desired with no discomfort whatsoever. On the contrary, it always leaves me feeling revitalized and invigorated. There is a very good physiological reason for that which I will share with you shortly, but first I have to relate my experience to you with my pinched nerve situation.

Obviously I had extremely high hopes of enjoying at least some measure of relief with my back; any relief at all would have been enthusiastically wel-comed. To my ecstatic astonishment after only my **very first time** on the table the nerve was released, the pain stopped, and from that day in early 2001 until today I have not had so much as a single twinge in my back let alone that feeling of being jabbed with an ice pick that I had to endure more often than not. As far as I was concerned it was nothing short of a miracle that freed me and allowed me to start to enjoy life again. You know how sometimes people ask if you were stranded on a deserted island and you could have only one thing with you what it would be? For me it would be my Inversion Table.

If you think about it, gravity is always pulling everything down and that goes for our body and every-thing in it. It's easy to see how the vertebrae in the spine can compress over time putting pressure on those ever-so-sensitive nerves. Regularly reversing the pull of gravity by going upside down and gently open-ing up and separating the vertebrae, even minutely, can only help reduce stress on the spine. Keeping the vertebrae evenly spaced relieves tension on the nerves and on the discs, or shock absorbers, that are between the vertebrae. I have even heard of people saying they have actually gained as much as a full inch in height from regularly going upside down.

Today I go upside down every day without fail for about four or five minutes; that's all it takes to maintain my spine and to prevent my vertebrae from going out of alignment or compressing down on a nerve. Some days I go for longer or do a few minutes two or three times a day simply because it leaves me feeling so good afterward. The reason why it feels so good is because of the increased flow of oxygenated blood to the brain, which in turn causes every activity of the body to function more effectively. Plus! Going upside down accelerates and improves the flow of lymph fluid throughout the body thereby intensifying and facilitating the accumulation and removal of toxins. I simply can't say enough good things about the value of using an Inversion Table to regularly go upside down. If you would like more information on obtaining the Teeter Inversion Table I use, you may call toll-free 877-335-1509 or go to our website: www.fitforlifetime.com.

As an interesting anecdote, a few months ago I ran into an acquaintance of mine that I had not seen for several months. The last time I saw him before that he was walking as though every step was agony and his face definitely gave the same impression. He looked transformed; like a new man. His entire demeanor was that of someone overwhelmingly happy just to be alive. We had barely finished our hellos before he blurted out with unbridled enthusiasm, "Harv, have you ever heard of an Inversion Table?" After telling him that I had, and that it changed my life, he told me that a bulging disc in his spine had nearly crippled him with unbearable pain. Someone told him about Inversion Tables, and like me, he immediately obtained one which relieved him of the pain almost overnight. He told me that he spends nearly two hours a day upside down because he loves the way it makes him feel.

Six. The beauty of adhering to the principles of eating designed to cleanse the connective tissue of toxins is that as far as the body is concerned it wants **all** toxins removed no matter where they may be concentrated. It doesn't matter if they are in the connective tissue, in the blood vessels in the head, in the colon, in an organ; anywhere they are, the effort to remove them never ceases. So long as sufficient energy is available, it is used to gather up and remove toxins from every corner of the body as quickly and efficiently as possible. That is why so many different ailments are simultaneously improved upon when a person eats more living food and unleashes the lymph system to perform its job.

There is a perfect example of what I am talking about that stands out in my memory. Several years ago a gentleman who lived in my neighborhood asked me if I would consider helping him with a problem that was, in his words, slowly sapping the life out of him. A problem with his colon that started out as a mild, intermittent annoyance had turned into a full blown, daily torment. He had been told by various doctors that he had spastic colon, colitis, irritable bowel syndrome, or possibly Crohn's disease for which there is supposedly "no known cause". He was regularly taking anti-inflammatory drugs however his situation continued to progressively worsen. He was practically unable to leave home out of fear of an "embarrassing episode" in public. When he started to see blood in his stool with greater regularity he became fearful of it culminating into colon cancer.

Needless to say this man was highly motivated and ready to try some alternative approach to the treatment he was receiving which was bringing him no relief whatsoever; not only no relief but the situation was actually worsening. Something different had to be done and he knew it. I explained to him essentially what I have put forth in this book to you about how connective tissue can become overburdened with uneliminated toxins. The difference was that it was his colon and not his connective tissue that was being affected. The solution, however, is the same.

Long story short, he put into practice the very principles I shared with you earlier and he followed them implicitly. The bleeding stopped completely in less than two weeks. Over the next few months he felt increasingly better with significantly less pain and discomfort. In less than six months he had no symptoms whatsoever, was not taking the anti-inflammatory drugs, and was feeling better than he had in nearly two years. It's difficult to put into words the genuine thankfulness this man had for the information that rescued him from what he thought was going to be his ultimate demise.

The part that tickled me was when he called some time later to ask me if I thought it was possible if what he had done to overcome his colon problem had also had an effect on his high blood pressure (hypertension) or if it was just a coincidence that it too was better. He had been taking Inderal for ten years and during that time his blood pressure was never in the normal range; all the drugs did was keep it under control which is all they're designed to do. But after six months of following the recommendations to help out with his colon problem he was no longer taking the Inderal and his blood pressure was in the normal range for the first time in ten years!

Plus! He told me that he had been dealing with psoriasis or eczema-like itchiness and flaking on the back of his neck for years and was forever rubbing various creams and lotions on it for relief but nothing ever did any good. It disappeared.

I'm beginning to feel like one of those commercials that keep saying, "But wait, there's more!" Additionally, he lost that "final 15 pounds" that so many people struggle with and he wasn't even trying to lose weight. It may appear on the surface to those who are unfamiliar with the nature of the body's healing dynamics that colitis, high blood pressure, itchy, flaky skin, and excess weight are four completely separate and distinct problems that require a specific treatment for each. However to the self-repairing, self-healing living body, all areas of distress are addressed equally and simultaneously.

My point in sharing this with you is to let you know that if the level of uneliminated toxins in your connective tissue has reached the point where you have Fibromyalgia, Lupus, or Arthritis, it's a pretty safe bet that there are some other, perhaps lesser painful, problems you are dealing with as well. I want you to know that as your body heals itself it will not stop at returning the connective tissue to its healthy state; it is not satisfied with correcting only some problems, it must of necessity correct any and all problems in the body and it will never stop striving to do so. Your only obligation is to see to it that you regularly supply the body with the energy it needs to get the job done.

Seven. I want to tell you about a sensational, totally natural product that will dramatically strengthen and nourish your body more so than any other product of its kind that I have ever seen. I have been using a "Green Superfood" on a daily basis since 1992, and I am certain that it has been instrumental in helping me maintain a high level of good health despite my challenges with

Agent Orange poisoning. I am convinced that you too will benefit from it no matter what health challenges you may be facing.

The last ten years has seen an explosion in the development of what are referred to as either, "Greens", "Green Drinks", or "Green Powders". This is an enormously encouraging trend that is helping offset the impact of the highly processed, denatured, devitalized, and acid-forming "food" that has unfortunately become standard fare for so many people. I made an exhaustive study of these products over the years and have found one that is, in my opinion, unparalleled. Not that there aren't others that are also very fine products, there are, but this is the one that stands out and appeals to me most because I am personally acquainted with the people responsible for bringing this product to market and am therefore familiar with their dedication to excellence.

The primary reason for my enthusiasm for this particular Green Superfood is the unwavering commitment to purity and superiority that is the trademark of every stage in the growing, harvesting, and formulation of the end product. There are no additives, fillers, or chemicals of any kind; **nothing** artificial. The ingredients are organically grown. It is packed with the vitamins, minerals, antioxidants, phytonutrients, amino acids, fatty acids, and plant-based enzymes that make it a truly **whole, living food**. One daily serving fills the requirement for nutrients equivalent to six cups of organic vegetables. It is a well known fact that disease proliferates in an acid environment. Green Superfoods neutralize acid and properly balance the acid-alkaline pH balance of the body.

All animal life on Earth, including human life, depends directly or indirectly on the plant kingdom for its very survival. Green Superfoods are really the ultimate health foods, for they are easily assimilated and highly concentrated in a rich blend of quality nutrients.

A well-documented study with people suffering with Rheumatoid Arthritis showed significant improvement after using a Green Superfood.[49A]

I am in the position, due to my condition of peripheral neuropathy, of having to be ultravigilant about what I put into my body. The dioxin poisoning has made me especially sensitive and susceptible to anything of an inferior or harmful nature. Fresh fruit and their juices, and Green Superfoods are the two most vital and important components of my diet and are responsible more than any other factor for the continued good health I enjoy today despite being poisoned by the deadliest chemical ever formulated. I thank the powers that be everyday that I have been fortunate enough to learn the unparalleled importance of dominating my diet with living food, especially fruit, and for a pristine, health promoting Green Superfood.

To find out more about **FEELING FIT GREENS** you may call toll-free 877-335-1509 or go to our website: www.fitforlifetime.com.

Eight. The most enduring image of humanity's exploration of space has turned out to be the sight of a small blue pearl of a planet orbiting a rather ordinary star in an out-of-the-way corner of the galaxy. From space, the blue color of our planet distinguishes it from anything else as far as our telescopes can see. The Hubble telescope can take pictures literally trillions of miles in any direction and our little blue pearl is the only one in sight.

What is it that makes our planet so unique, special, and extraordinary? Water. Water not only colors our world but also provides it with the capacity to harbor life. Water is Nature's catalyst; the key to life. There are places on Earth that are so dry, parched, and inhospitable looking that you would think no life could possibly be sustained there. Then along comes a life-giving rain and a dazzling spectacle of transformation occurs. In only a few short days there is a lush carpet of plants and flowers in a circus of colors as far as the eye can see where only a few days earlier there was nothing but parched and cracked earth. Animals by the thousands seem to appear out of nowhere to feast on the bounty.

Recognizing the uniqueness of our planet and the primary role water plays in our life, and in our health, can only rightly cause us to view water in a new, more reverential way. When we honor the miraculous experience of our life, we must acknowledge the incalculable importance of water and strive to grasp the full measure of the fundamental role it plays in our health and our fitness.

In the same way that water is the key to life and the health of our planet, it is also a primary key to our personal health and well-being. In seeking vibrant health for ourselves and our loved ones, we would be well advised to educate ourselves about water. And aided by a new advanced technology and water science, it has been discovered that water is not "just water" anymore. A new class and generation of advanced hydration and nutritional waters have been designed to take us beyond simply surviving, to actually thriving as fit, healthy, high performance individuals. These discoveries will have a profound effect on our national and global health in the years to come.

In looking at our blue planet it quickly becomes apparent that most of the surface of the planet is water, in fact about 70% of it is water. I don't know why it is called planet Earth, when clearly it should be called planet Water. A most interesting fact to ponder is that our bodies are also approximately 70% water. We are, in the most literal sense possible, water beings living on a water planet. Our body fluids are an internal ocean that regulates and drives all body functions in the same way that water and water cycles govern organic life on Earth.

As we all make our way through this journey called life, there is no gift that is more desired or more cherished than the gift of good health. Some might say that monetary wealth is most desired but, as I asked earlier, what good is a lot of money if you're too sick to enjoy it? Health is the greatest of gifts and it is impossible to discuss the subject without also discussing the role of water in acquiring and maintaining our health. No more than one could discuss the nature of a majestic 200 foot redwood tree without also discussing the soil in which it grows.

In striving for the highest level of health that can be attained, it is instructive to know that the two most extensive systems in the living body work hand-in-hand with one another in a never-ending, never-tiring effort to keep the body as healthy as is possible. The first is the cardiovascular system, which has at its center the heart, pumping six quarts of blood through an amazing 90,000 miles of blood vessels bringing oxygen to every cell of the body. The extreme importance of keeping the entire cardiovascular system in top working condition is evidenced by the fact that cardiovascular disease takes more lives than all other causes of death by disease **combined**.

The second, as has already been discussed at length is the lymph system; the heart and soul of the immune system. As you now know, the body is constantly generating wastes, referred to as toxins, both from the billions of spent cells that die off every day and from the residue of the some 70 tons of food we will each eat in our lifetime. If these toxins were allowed to be produced in our body unchecked, we would quickly be ushered to the grave, and they are the underlying cause of Fibromyalgia, Lupus, Arthritis, and Chronic Fatigue Syndrome. It is the job of the lymph system which contains three times more lymph fluid than the body does blood to see to it that that never happens by gathering up these toxins from every cell everywhere in the body, breaking them down, and removing them.

It is the activities of the cardiovascular system and the lymph system that determines how long we will live and how healthy we will be. No matter what one's health goals are, to lose weight, increase energy, remove pain, overcome or prevent disease—whatever—you can be absolutely certain beyond even the most infinitesimal uncertainty that **nothing** will be achieved without the constant and tireless effort of the cardiovascular and lymph systems. Of that there is **no doubt**.

"What," you may be asking, "do the cardiovascular system and lymph system have to do with the discussion of water?" Just this: the blood that fuels the cardiovascular system and the lymph fluid that fuels the lymph system are 90% water! And it doesn't stop there. The activities of the cardiovascular and lymph systems, and the **trillions** of other activities performed by the living body every moment, are all overseen by and conducted by what is considered to be the most complex and astonishing creation in all of nature: the human brain. The brain is 85% water, as is the cerebrospinal fluid that cushions the brain. So is the amniotic fluid that envelopes and protects a fetus. Saliva is almost all water and without it our tongue would stick to the inside of our mouth; we wouldn't be able to swallow. The fluid that moistens the eye so it can move with ease, as well as tears, both mostly water. If not for water, food would not be digested as digestive juices are practically all water.

The entire process of bringing nutrients **to** the cells and removing wastes from the cells is dependent upon water as the transport medium. The fluid that surrounds all the internal organs of the body is made up of water and without it the organs would stick together and tear. And of course, the connective tissue is also mostly water. All the joints of the body move with such ease because of synovial fluid which is 90% water and without it the joints quickly become susceptible to Arthritis. Even our bones are 35% water. **We are water beings!**

Remove all water from the human body and what is left would fit into a shoebox. When you consider that water is the second most urgent and necessary requirement in order to stay alive, second only to air, it's rather shocking how few people fully recognize the truly devastating repercussions to the body when insufficiently hydrated, and conversely, the immeasurable good that is the result of properly meeting all of the body's water needs.

It's surprising how few people realize how much water is actually lost from the body every day. As water beings on a water planet the human body is constructed so that there is an unceasing, round-the-clock ebb and flow of water into and out of the body. Every day each one of us loses about two quarts of water. Depending upon certain variables such as physical activity and diet, it can easily be **twice** that amount. Water is lost through both perspiration and respiration.

Our skin contains millions of pores, all of which are **always** secreting a certain amount of moisture. Obviously when exercise or physical activity is heightened we perspire more heavily and can clearly see the loss of water, but there is not a moment, day or night, that our skin is not excreting some water. We also lose water every time we exhale. Breathe on a mirror or window and you can actually see the moisture from your lungs on the glass. Since you exhale many thousands of times a day, each and every time you do you lose some water.

This water **must be replaced every day** and failing to do so will cause you more harm than you could possibly imagine. Depriving the body of its water needs, intentionally or unintentionally, can have catastrophic results that negatively affect every activity and function of the living body. No matter what your health goals are, **all** are sabotaged by short changing the body of its water needs.

I have been studying and teaching the principles of a healthy lifestyle for 35 of my 60 years on Earth. I have seen many ironies relating to people's quest to live a pain free life dominated by health and well-being. I can tell you from my experiences that perhaps the most tragic irony of all is the one associated with the pain, ill health, and disease that afflicts so many people who could have avoided it all if only they had done something as simple and natural as properly hydrating their body.

Millions of people continue to scramble around trying all manner of remedies in order to recapture or maintain their health. They resort to drugs which are inherently toxic and dangerous and all too frequently even kill. They take fistfuls of supplements, most of which are synthesized in a laboratory or extracted with chemicals or heat, which in either case compromise their worth. They go on fad diets that are only temporary at best and stress the body. And of course there is no shortage of expensive treatments all designed to try and force the body into doing what it would have automatically done for itself if only it wasn't sabotaged due to insufficient hydration.

For whatever reason, people have failed to recognize the immeasurable benefit they could reap simply by replenishing the water they lose every day which would properly hydrate their body. This **alone** would significantly optimize the body's own healing capabilities which would in turn dramatically improve a person's health and well-being.

I say this is tragic because even though there is something so natural and uncomplicated as simply providing the living body with the water it must have to survive, which would improve health, there are estimates that go as high as 75% of the population being under hydrated, many of them chronically. There are actually a significant number of people who drink no water at all. As embarrassed as I am to say it, there was a time in my early life when I was one of them. My attitude was, why drink water when I could have a Dr. Pepper instead? And believe me when I tell you that my health suffered as a result; even though I didn't know it at the time.

People have told me that instead of water they drink coffee, soda, or pasteurized bottled juices. What they don't realize is that they all are highly acidic in the body and counterproductive because they don't properly hydrate the cells. They drink these liquids instead of water and then wonder why they don't feel well and can't maintain their health.

Here is a totally obvious, simple, and straightforward approach to taking care of one's health, **the way**

Nature intended for us to, that of simply supplying the living body with the water it must have for its very survival, and for some inexplicable reason it is not being utilized. People actually deprive themselves of something, not only essential to life and health promoting, but also so easily accessible. It is the irony of ironies. I guess the old adage is true that the simplest solutions in life are the ones most frequently overlooked.

Research has shown that when body cells are properly hydrated, they become enlarged and trigger a healing mechanism. This healing mechanism is the result of such factors as a reduction of cellular acidity, increased fat burning, and repair of DNA. It has further been demonstrated that when the body becomes **de**hydrated, the cells become deflated and trigger the opposite of healing, or sickness, in the cells. This begins with a buildup of cellular acid and toxins which leads to oxygen starvation and acceleration of the aging process.

Viewed from the perspective of one's health being significantly impacted by whether or not body cells are properly and sufficiently hydrated, we all need to be ever concerned about the quality and quantity of the water we drink. As water beings on the water planet it is only logical to make this a high priority in our life. We have come a long way from the days when I was a kid when if you wanted a glass of water you simply went to the kitchen sink and drank your fill. Today, I'm sorry to say, that much of the nation's groundwater and underground aquifers are contaminated with unhealthy levels of chemicals.

Today, my attitude is, drink **anything** but tap water. I don't care who says what about how pure or how clean commercial "purified" tap water is, I wouldn't drink tap water unless there was absolutely no choice. Many people drink tap water without so much as giving it a second thought. All manner of chemicals are added to water at purification plants, and that water picks up metallic contaminants merely by flowing through the intricate web of pipelines, some of which are decades old, before reaching you. Almost all such water contains such chemical pollutants. A host of chemicals, wastes, agricultural fertilizers, and industrial pollutants all find their way into the water supply. To counteract this, other chemicals are deliberately added to the water supply to "purify" it and kill bacteria.

We are most fortunate to be living in an era when technological advancements in water science have progressed to a staggering degree. Most people are not even remotely aware of accomplishments that have been achieved in making available water that is infinitely superior to anything that has ever been available in the past. Water is most definitely not "just water" any more. In only a few short years we have progressed from the need to filter our basic tap water, to the need to purify our water, all the way to effectively enhancing our water to bring about maximum benefit.

I've heard people say, "Water is water, what difference does it make?" That simply is not accurate. In the same way there is pure and clean air, and air that is polluted; and food that is fresh and wholesome and food that is over processed and unhealthy, there is water that is far superior to other water. In studying hydration, scientists have determined that water and hydration may be adequate around the **outside** of the cell, but without the right kind of water with the right electrical/mineral mix, and proper surface tension, water flow **into** the cells is ineffective. The result is cellular dehydration.

Today, owing in large part to the advancements in water science and technology there is a dizzying array of waters available on the market, including well water, bottled water, filtered water, purified water, spring water, artesian water, mineral water, distilled water, soft water, hard water, deionized water, electrolyzed water, and structured water.

With so many waters on the market the questions begging to be asked are, "How do I choose the right water?" "How do I know which water is best?" "How can I be sure the water I'm drinking is what it is advertised to be?" "How can I tell if my water meets the highest standards available?" These are legitimate questions that anyone concerned with good health should be interested in having satisfactorily answered. They are most certainly the issues with which I personally want to be comfortable. Especially in light of the fact that there **are** going to be waters advertised and sold as superior which plainly are not.

That image of the clear mountain spring on the label may be misleading. Contrary to popular belief, bottled water isn't always cleaner and safer than tap water. According to the New York based environmental advocacy group, the National Resources Defense Council, about 1/3 of the 100 brands of bottled water it tested violated stringent state and federal purity standards.[50] CNN reported that they had four bottled waters taken at random off the shelf and independently tested to see if they were everything they were advertised to be. Three out of four were not![51]

I struggle with these issues the same as you. I am deeply concerned about my health and I want to be certain I am drinking **only** the very best water available anywhere, period! Knowing as I do the overwhelming importance of properly hydrating the cells of my body and the immeasurable good that is the result of doing so, I refuse to compromise even to the slightest degree when it comes to my drinking water. In the same way I know there are drinking waters that are not as good as they are advertised to be, I also know there have to be ones that are of the highest quality possible. I am always on the lookout for the most cutting edge, up-to-date, finest water available and I am ever so pleased to tell you that I have found one that I consider to be the "Rolls Royce" of bottled waters.

I mentioned earlier that my decision to attach my name to a product is not something I do hastily. I am not a product driven person—I won't endorse just anything for the sake of a check. Instead, I endorse and promote only a very select few; only ones that I am absolutely certain are of the highest quality and benefit for people who put their trust in me to lead them in the right direction. If I am not willing to consume a product myself I would **never** recommend it to others, no matter what I was offered to do so.

In the mid 1980s when the first **FIT FOR LIFE** book was released I drank, and highly recommended distilled water. That was before many of the technological water science advancements in existence today had been made and I felt distilled was the best way to go at the time. Not that there is anything wrong with drinking distilled water, there isn't, it is infinitely superior to regular tap water; no comparison. But as knowledge increased and advancements were made even more superior waters became available. At the close of the 1990s I recommended one of those that I found to be excellent which has gone through some name changes but remains an outstanding water. As time moves forward, more is learned and more is able to be achieved in water science; one must at all the time be on the alert and be flexible and ready to recognize a superior product when it comes along. I am always on that alert and will continue to pass on to you anything I feel will help you in your efforts.

Today the water that has captured my attention and which I am convinced is the ultimate, most advanced drinking water on the market, and the one I have decided to drink exclusively is called **Penta**. Backed up by some very impressive science, Penta's ultra-premium, purified drinking water is, in my opinion, the very best of the best. The people who are responsible for bringing this water to the marketplace have an unflinching dedication to excellence and it is what fuels their uncompromising effort to have the quintessential water in the industry. It only has to be tasted and experienced to see that it is something special. There are several factors that make **Penta** the exceptional drinking water that it is.

Penta is the purest known bottled drinking water on the market, and is the top-selling bottled water item in health food stores. The water undergoes a rigorous 13-step purification process in a state-of-the-art bottling facility. This process—**which far exceeds FDA standards for bottled water**—is designed to remove every possible natural and human made bacteriological and mineral impurity, pollutant or contaminant found in water, including bad tastes, odor, arsenic, bacteria, chlorine, chromium 6, fluoride, lead, and pesticides. These impurities have been found in other drinking water, but have never been found in **Penta**.

No chemicals are ever used to purify the water. At the end of the 13-step purification process, the total dissolved solids (that's the bad stuff you do **not** want in the water) will average less than 0.5 parts per million (regular water is 550!)—making **Penta** the purest known bottled water on the market (even purer than distilled water). The water undergoes a patented physics process using high-energy sound waves that gives it many unique properties. This proprietary technology, known as the "Penta Process," actually changes the structure of the water making it the only bottled water that uses physics, not chemicals, to restructure its water. It takes about 11 hours to make a single bottle of **Penta** water.

Let's face it, in the final analysis what is of greatest importance, aside from the unsurpassed purity of the water itself is the ability for it to hydrate the cells. Because minerals in drinking water can slow or even inhibit the cellular absorption of water, ultra-purified water like Penta is ideal for optimal hydration. Many do not drink enough water because they don't like the taste of water. However, Penta makes it easy to stay properly hydrated because of its ultraclean taste.

One cannot help but be impressed with the well documented, peer reviewed scientific studies that bear out what is stated here about **Penta** water and which can be reviewed at the company's web site. There are also numerous testimonials from people in all walks of life. I was most impressed with some of the professional athletes, as well as health and fitness experts, who now swear by the water and have made it their water of choice; also available for review.

I have always been enormously impressed with triathletes. I don't know how they do it; first a two mile swim, then they jump on their bikes and go full out for 112 miles, then run a full 26.2 mile marathon, with competitors giving it their all to do it faster than anyone else. I get winded just writing about it. You know those people are looking for any kind of competitive edge they can possibly find, and proper hydration has to be right on top of the list of musts.

In October 2001, a study was completed at the University of St. Thomas Department of Health and Human Performance in St. Paul, Minnesota, which demonstrated a significant increase in athletic performance, as measure for power, endurance and speed after drinking **Penta** water for three days. Eight competitive triathletes and/or cyclists were tested and the results, if translated to actual competition, would reflect substantial improvement (up to 15% decrease in overall time) for each athlete after consumption of **Penta** water.

I know that anyone can say anything they want about a product and how good it is, and quite frankly, how would you know if what you were hearing or reading was accurate or not? But the thing is, amongst the glut of inferior foods, waters, and nutritionals that are regularly advertised and promoted there has to be those select, elite ones that are everything they are purported to be. It is my experience that **Penta** is one of those.

Be that as it may, what I would ask of anyone reading this right now is not to simply take my word for what I'm saying, no matter how promising it may sound; but rather to do what I and many others have done and that is to see for yourself. Think of the improvement in your health and life that is possible if what I've told you here is valid, sound, and true. Fortunately the result of properly hydrating your body with an extremely pure, high quality water proves itself in a relatively short period of time.

I would ask that you drink, to the exclusion of any other water, at least two liters of **Penta** a day for two weeks and see if you don't notice a definite and recognizable difference in your well-being. There are numerous examples of others whose only lifestyle change was to improve the hydration of their body by taking this challenge who have realized a marked improvement in their health and well-being. Some of the transformations of which I speak are truly remarkable and awe inspiring. The parent company has these testimonials on file.

The term miraculous has been used to describe some of the improvements people have experienced. To be sure, the water merits being mentioned in terms of these improvements but I want to be sure you realize that the water itself is not what healed; rather it is the supreme hydrating qualities of the water that enabled the living body to unleash its own inherent and unrivaled healing capabilities. When this unsurpassed healing mechanism of the body is brought to bear, the results can indeed appear miraculous.

Water is simply too important a factor in a person's health to not do whatever is necessary to seek out and consume the very finest available. Whether attempting to overcome ill health or to maintain one's good health, properly hydrating the cells can only increase one's chances of success. Without a doubt, those desirous of overcoming Fibromyalgia, Lupus, Arthritis, or Chronic Fatigue Syndrome, absolutely **must** pay as much attention to the water they drink as they do to the food they eat. Don't shortchange yourself, when it comes to the water you drink and you will be glad for the remainder of your healthy and fit life. To learn more about **Penta** water or to find out how to obtain it, you may call toll-free 877-335-1509 or go to our website: www.fitforlifetime.com.

CHAPTER NINE

YOU ARE
WHAT YOU THINK
YOU ARE

Well, there you have it. I have done my level best to show you how to conquer pain and overcome Fibromyalgia, Lupus, Arthritis, and Chronic Fatigue Syndrome. The rest is up to you. I have done my part and your body will most definitely do its part; now it's time for you to do yours. Before I sign off I wish to discuss one last area of importance that, although frequently overlooked, plays a significant role in overcoming Fibromyalgia, Lupus, Arthritis, and Chronic Fatigue Syndrome, or any other ailment of the body for that matter. Some people are convinced that it plays the biggest role of all.

I have discussed at great length the effect that diet and water have on the health of the body. In no way can they be minimized. Of equal importance is another aspect of your diet—your mental diet. You feed your mind with thoughts the same way you feed your body with food. Volumes have been written on the mind-body connection and the extent to which the mind impacts the body either positively or negatively, depending on the nature of one's thoughts. There are numerous, well documented studies showing over and over how people have both made themselves sick and made themselves well as a result of the thoughts that dominated their thinking.

In the physical world that we relate to with our five senses, it's well known that there are natural laws that are simple and unyielding. The classic example has to do with the planting of seeds in the ground. If an orchard is planted with orange seeds, when harvest time comes there will be lots of oranges. Plant thistle seeds, and come harvest time don't expect oranges, because all there will be are thistles. Now you might be saying, "Gee, you don't say? Tell me something I **don't** know." Yes, that is as obvious as saying the sun is hot, but what is not as obvious to some people is that the mind is as fertile as is soil, and the law of sowing and reaping is just as unyielding in the mental world as in the physical. In other words, thoughts are like seeds in that they become things as surely as seeds become plants.

Even though the effect that thoughts and the mind can have on physical health has been known for hundreds if not thousands of years, the people who "don't know" have notoriously discounted the idea that the mind can help heal the body. In 1990 the American Medical Association surveyed its members and found that only a paltry 10% believed in the mind-body connection.[52] How supposedly "educated and intelligent" people could be so in the dark on the subject is mind-boggling to me. Especially considering that studies from their own journals and textbooks have shown it to be so. It would be like saying that apples on a tree have no connection to the soil in which the tree grows.

In one long-term university level study pertaining to optimism and pessimism, it showed that, across the board, pessimists died before optimists. Those who ranked within the top 25% as the most negative had the highest death rate. In contrast, the death rate of those who ranked as the most optimistic was less than one-half that of pessimists.[53]

One ten-year study on elderly people showed that those who actually thought of themselves and labeled themselves as old or elderly had a significantly higher death rate over the course of the study than those who thought of themselves as middle-aged.[54])

There are enough studies to fill this book several times over that show the power of the mind to affect the body. Thousands of them. Some of the most impressive and convincing evidence comes from what is referred to as the "placebo effect." To determine the effectiveness of a drug, a group of people with a certain illness is divided into two groups. One group receives the drug, and the other receives the placebo, usually a coated sugar pill. Neither group knows which it has received.

Time and again it has been shown that 30% to 60% report relief of pain, even stabbing pain, from the placebo.[55] The mind is so powerful in producing whatever reality it is convinced of that up to 50% of the subjects in some studies actually exhibit side effects from the placebo.[56] In one astonishing case involving the testing of an antihistamine, the subjects receiving the placebos actually experienced more side effects than those who received the medication![57]

In one startling study of a new kind of chemotherapy, 30% of those in the control group, the group given placebos, **lost their hair.**[58] Such is the power of the mind when it's convinced of a certain outcome. This is pretty powerful stuff, wouldn't you agree? This awesome power resides in you right now, and you can use it any time you want in any way you want.

Perhaps you are familiar with the work of Bernie S. Siegel, M.D. He received worldwide notoriety as a result of showing people how to use their mind to send positive messages of love and healing to their body to overcome even catastrophic cases of disease. In his enormously successful book, *Love, Medicine and Miracles*, he wrote, "Many of the mind's effects are achieved directly on the body's tissues without any awareness on our part. The body responds to the mind's messages whether conscious or unconscious."

I could easily quote dozens of examples of comments made by great and respected individuals all throughout history who made comments similar to Dr. Siegel's. Two of my favorites come from Buddha, who said, "All that we are is the result of what we have thought," and Jesus, who said over and over in so many different ways, "It is done unto you as you believe."

Every great thinker the world has ever known has made reference to the untapped power our thoughts have, when properly channeled, to positively affect our life. Let's say, for the sake of argument, that they are right. Let's say that Dr. Siegel, Buddha, Jesus, and the long list of others who made similar comments were right on target.

There's something we all do during our waking hours. It's called "self-speak." We're always talking to ourselves, either out loud or in our head. "Don't forget to pick up the dry cleaning." "What am I going to do with myself today?" "Why don't you stop wasting so much time?" "When are you going to get serious about exercise?" "How long are you going to put up with so-and-so?" "Boy, am I tired." And on and on it goes.

Sometimes our self-speak is used to either berate or congratulate ourselves. "What's wrong with me? Why can't I ever catch a break?" "Way to go! That's how to close that deal." "I'm never going to get ahead. I must have been born under a bad star." "All right! That's more like it. I knew I could do it." "You're such a loser." "You're the best!"

My point with all of this is, since we're already thinking **something** about ourselves, why not go on the premise that what we think consistently will become a reality in our life? If that's the case and negative thoughts will bring negative results and positive thoughts will bring positive results, it just makes good common sense to send positive messages to ourselves. Positive thoughts will never bring about negative results, but negative thoughts surely might, so why take a chance?

Which of the two following statements repeated over and over to yourself do you think will empower and uplift you, and which do you think will not?

"I don't know why I should even try anymore. It doesn't do any good."

"I'm the child of a loving God that **wants** me to be happy and fulfilled."

I'll bet I can guess which one Buddha and Jesus would prefer. The human mind is the great gift that separates us from the rest of the animal kingdom. What is absolutely known about the mind is but a single drop of water compared to the ocean, which represents what is yet to be learned.

Whether you are self-speaking to yourself about overcoming Fibromyalgia, Lupus, Arthritis, and Chronic Fatigue Syndrome or any other health challenge, your relationships, your finances—whatever the subject, see if you can start to send only kind, non-judgmental, positive, uplifting, loving and empowering messages to yourself. Every time you do, you send that message to all the cells of your body, which are sensitive and receptive to the messages they receive. Soon you will realize that the universe is on your side; that the good thoughts you sow into the great unknown turn into the harvest of good you reap in your life.

Believe me, I know from experience what a challenge it is to wake up in the morning feeling poorly and launching into a rendition of, "Isn't life grand?" But I also know from experience that believing in my heart that the pain is a temporary condition and that better times are coming, reaps benefits in the long run. Even if at first you have to force yourself to think positively, do it. There simply is no time, no matter what the circumstances, that negative thinking is more advantages than positive thinking. It doesn't work that way.

As you start to use the information you have learned in this book and begin to feel better and healthier, it will become easier and easier to maintain a positive outlook on everything in your life. Have faith. Believe in yourself. Trust that the powers that be are in your corner. And let me hear from you. I'd like to know how you're doing.

In all areas of your life, may God bless your every breath and guide your every step.

A MESSAGE
FROM THE AUTHOR

Perhaps you are familiar with the phrase "Often imitated—never duplicated." The name **FIT FOR LIFE** was coined for the ideas and book I co-wrote in 1985. Over the years, as **FIT FOR LIFE** gained notoriety, the name has been used by a number of entities with which I have no personal connection.

I would like to assure you of my continued interest in hearing from you with any questions, comments, or experiences you may have as a result of reading this book.

In addition, to order or obtain more information about products, services, or newsletter, the official contact points for me are as follows:

Postal Address:

Harvey Diamond

P.O. Box 811, Osprey, Florida 34229

Website:

www.fitforlifetime.com

E-mail:

info@fitforlifetime.com

Fax:

305-723-6166

PRODUCTS:

Live Plant Digestive Enzymes, Coral Calcium, Green Superfood, Champion Juicer,

REBOUND*AIR* Rebounder,

Teeter Inversion Table, **Penta** Water

The full line of **Enzymedica** products may be obtained at the best independent health food stores in the country. You will also find them at such national chains as Whole Foods and Wild Oats.

Enzymedica is the manufacturer and distributor of some of the highest quality plant based enzyme products available anywhere. With knowledge that there are a number of enzyme supplement products to chose from, Enzymedica products stand alone for the following reasons:

- Enzymedica uses an exclusive *Thera-blend* process for its protease, lipase, amylase and cellulase. This means that each of these enzymes actually represents multiple strains. For example, there are actually four proteases in the *Thera-blend* protease. They are blended for their ability to break down more protein, fats and carbohydrates over a longer time period in the body.

- Enzymedica products contain the *highest therapeutic activities* available. No other company uses such high active units in a multiple enzyme line. In addition to a digestive enzyme (Digest) that is on average six times stronger than their competitors, Enzymedica has a therapeutic digestive enzyme blend (Digest Gold), a high amylase (V- Gest), a high protease (Virastop), and a high lipase (Lypo) product. These are the only ones of their kind.

- All of Enzymedica products are **100%** vegan and vegetarian

- Enzymedica uses *no fillers* in any of its enzyme formulations. You will no doubt notice how small the capsules Enzymedica uses are in comparison to similar products. This is a result of using concentrates with no fillers.

- Enzymedica's entire focus and purpose is enzymes. They are **the experts**. Unlike most of their competitors, Enzymedica does not make vitamin supplements. All they manufacture is the highest quality, highest potency enzyme products available.

- Enzymedica has every batch **third party tested**. This ensures they always meet label claim.

- Enzymedica products are **Health Professional proven**. They utilize the expertise of doctors, clinicians and health professionals in all of their formulations. In addition to the Enzymedica line of enzymes, they also manufacture and distribute Theramedix, a health professional version of Enzymedica products.

I've been asked about nutritional supplements for well over 30 years. Along with some of the most accomplished nutritionists, scientists, and doctors we have assembled a group of products of the highest quality available that provide abundant amounts of every nutrient essential for life. The **FEELING FIT FOUR** kit includes the following:

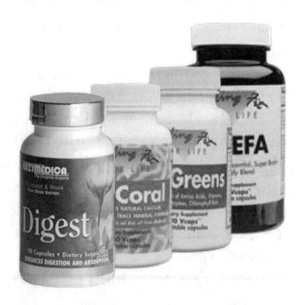

• **Digest 90 Vcaps**

Highly effective live plant enzymes, supporting digestion of protein, carbohydrates and fats. Relieves gas
and bloating. Formulated without fillers or toxic excipients like magnesium stearate. Encapsulated in 100%
Vegan approved vegetable capsules. Take before every
meal that contains cooked food to help conserve your
precious supply of life-giving enzymes.

• **LifeCoral 60 Vcaps**

Highly alkaline coral minerals with potent mycleial
mushroom extract for an ideal, alkaline pH. Contains
the best minerals found on earth. 100% pure Japanese
coral minerals: highly ionized calcium, magnesium (an
ideal 2:1 ratio) along with trace minerals. Coupled
with speical mycelial mushroom extract to provide
herbal vitamin D. Vitamin D is esssential for transport
of calcium into cells. No synthetics or fillers.
LifeCoral is the perfect source of the calcium and other
minerals necessary to keep bones and body systems
strong and healthy.

• **LifeGreens 90 Vcaps**

World-class greens for optimal health. Contains grade
10, non-hybrid cereal grasses -- abundant in healing
agents. Contains every known vitamin, mineral and
enzyme essential to life. Quantum breakthrough in
intracellular nourishment and DNA repair. No toxic
excipients, like magnesium stearate, are found in this

Vegan approved product. LifeGreens contain biologically available nutrients that provide unmatched protection for organs, glands, skin, eyes and bones.

• **LifeEFA 120 Vcaps**

World-class, life-essential super brain & body oils. Premier source of essential fatty acids using an ideal ratio of GLA, Omega 3, 6 & 9 fatty acids. Beyond organic, cold pressed, unrefined, solvent-free oils: Flax, Moroccan Olive, English Borage and Sesame oils. Encapsulated in 100% pure, preservative free vegetable capsules which dissolve rapidly and are easily digested. LifeEFA is a result of careful clinical measurement of essential fatty acids needed to correct the imbalance of fats in the typical American diet.

For information or a catalog on the full line of Feeling Fit products,

Call toll free:

877-942-4492 or 877-215-1212

Or visit our Website www.fitforlifetime.com

~ *Special Note* ~

On a very limited, first come, first serve basis, Harvey will be making himself available for personal phone consultations. To find out how to schedule your one hour, one-on-one phone consultation with Harvey, and to make arrangements for payment, please send an e-mail to hd@hdffl.com.

ENZYMES FOR LIFE

You are probably familiar with the expression, "Big things come in small packages." If that saying is true, then I want to tell you about one of the biggest little packages I've ever seen. In only a few short pages, you're going to learn about an astonishingly simple tool that, without exaggeration, will be one of the most profound and effective means by which you ensure for yourself that long, pain-free life that has been referred to throughout this book.

At public seminars I have given over the last twenty-five years or so, one question I always ask my audiences to respond to by raising their hands is, "How many people here love to eat?" Without fail, all in attendance throw their hands skyward as though they were reaching up to snatch hundred-dollar bills out of the air that have fallen from the ceiling. Many thrust

both hands in the air with such enthusiasm you'd think
I just asked them "How many people here would like
a brand-new car of their choice, for free?" When the
audiences were large, a thousand people or more, the
upraised arms looked like a flock of flamingos coming
in for a landing on the Serengeti Plain. After the flut-
tering and laughter subsided, I would explain what I
have spoken of earlier: that each and every one of us
will consume some 70 tons of food in our lifetime. So
it certainly makes sense that if we're going to spend
the amount of time necessary to obtain and eat 70 tons
of food, we might just as well enjoy ourselves while
we're doing it. Don't you agree?

I have already made the point well how much energy is required for the digestive process. The entire pro-
gression of digestion and metabolism, the breaking
down of the 70 tons of food, extraction and utilization
of nutrients, and elimination of the wastes, will require
more energy in your lifetime than all other uses of
energy **combined**! Reflect on that for a while and you
are sure to be impressed.

The digestion of food takes a huge amount of your
energy, more than for anything else you do, which is
why you are tired after a meal. And the bigger the
meal, the more tired you are. People tire after eating
because the digestive process demands the expenditure of such a high amount of energy.

You know, from the time you are born until the time you leave this life, you have a certain amount of life energy available to you. When it's gone, life is over. Since it is an unassailable, physiological fact that more of that energy will be used up for the digestive process than all other uses combined, does it not seem prudent beyond measure for you to make use of any possible means by which to either streamline the digestive process or in some manner reduce its burden? To me, the answer to that question is more obvious than the answer to the question: "Is the sun hot?" Reducing the burden of the digestive process can have but one long-term effect: It will improve the length and quality of your life. There's simply no doubt about that.

All my books delineate methods you can use to decrease the work of the digestive process, to give it periodic rests; my ideas emphasize how important it is for you not to push the digestive process beyond its capabilities. I know many of you reading this right now have read FIT FOR LIFE, and that makes me extremely happy. And I know that there are those of you who have not read it. (We know who you are, incidentally.) FIT FOR LIFE contains an entire section on proper food combining, an approach that has many benefits. Food combining is a way to optimize energy from the digestive tract by not mixing protein (such as meat) with starches (such as potatoes or rice). The

Number 1 benefit of the practice, as I explained earlier, is that it streamlines digestion. In **this** book, periodic Mono-dieting shows you how to free a significant amount of energy from the digestive process which is, in turn, used by the body to thoroughly clean the lymph system; this ultimately prevents disease in the long term while dramatically improving all aspects of health in the short term including overcoming pain.

I regularly talk about the work of Dr. Roy Walford, a world renowned scientist who **doubled** the lifespan and **dramatically** improved the health of mice he experimented with merely by fasting and totally resting their digestive systems for two days a week. Animals in the wild or kept as pets will instinctively stop eating when they're sick or injured in order to free digestive energy for the healing process. And of course, children and adults also lose their appetite when they are "under the weather," which is, once again, the body's protective mechanism trying to divert to the healing process the energy that would be spent on digestion.

From what you have read so far, I'm certain that you see that **anything** you can do to reduce the work of your digestive system is an extremely wise thing to do. That being the case, I must say that I am astounded that one of the most simple, effective means by which anyone can immediately start to dramatically reduce the work of their digestive system, thereby ensuring a longer, healthier, more pain free life, is largely unknown to the vast majority of the population. In fact, I wonder if there is anything, anywhere that has the potential to do so much good that has been more overlooked and neglected. And what is this certain thing I am referring to? Enzymes!

To explain enzymes and what they do, I could launch into a convoluted, scientific dissertation about how amylase, which breaks down carbohydrates, splits starches into different disaccharides, or how pepsin, which works on proteins, splits proteins into smaller peptide chains, all so food can be broken down and made small enough to pass through the villi, the small pores of the intestines, and into the bloodstream. And if my goal was to cause you to skip this section, I would do just that. Instead, I wish to give you an ultra-simplified, totally non-technical explanation, to be certain that you fully grasp and recognize the immense, life-saving role enzymes play in your health. Anyone wishing a more detailed and scientific understanding of enzymes and their activity in the body can certainly read up on them. But my primary goal here is to leave you with a newfound sense of the enormity of the role enzymes fulfill in our daily lives.

Enzymes are tiny protein chemicals that carry an essential energy source needed for every chemical action and reaction that occurs in your body. We're talking about a number so immense you couldn't possibly comprehend it. Literally trillions upon trillions of chemical activities are taking place in your body right now. **None would occur without enzymes.** All life, plant or animal, requires enzymes to continue living. Enzymes **mean** life. Enzymes **are** life. Whenever you hear about or talk about your body doing something, anything, no matter what, that has anything whatsoever to do with the building, repairing, or maintaining of any part of your body, inside or out, enzymes are involved. And without them, nothing would get done. Life would cease to exist. The living body is under a great burden every day to produce the volume of enzymes necessary to run efficiently.

There are three classes of enzymes you need to be aware of. First are metabolic enzymes, which are referred to as the "body's labor force" because virtually every activity of your body depends upon them. Without these power-packed little dynamos continually at work, you couldn't swallow, blink your eyes, circulate blood, breathe in and out, transform food into blood and muscle and bone, walk, talk, or anything else. The activities of the lymph system and its role in keeping you well while preventing pain and disease is entirely dependent, as is every other function of the body, on metabolic enzymes!

We all know how exceedingly important it is to eat a good diet so that the full complement of nutrients— the vitamins, minerals, essential fatty acids, and amino acids—can be made available to the body to carry out all of its functions. But no matter how pure the diet, no matter how many high-quality nutrients are introduced into the body, it all means nothing without metabolic enzymes.

I'll use a simple analogy to explain why this is so. If you wished to build a house, you could bring to the site all the materials you need to build it: lumber, hammers, nails, cement, bricks, mortar, insulation, wiring, roofing material, everything. But just putting all the materials on the site won't create the house. Unless the construction workers show up to assemble all the materials, the house will not be built. No matter how plentiful the materials, no matter how high the quality of the materials, if there are no construction workers, there is no house. Metabolic enzymes are your body's "construction workers." Without them, nothing gets done, and I mean nothing.

Here is the single most important fact about metabolic enzymes that you must be aware of. There are a finite number of metabolic enzymes that can be produced by your body. I want to be absolutely certain you know exactly what I'm saying. Your body can produce a certain number of metabolic enzymes, and no more! You can, you **will**, run out of them! And there is a word to describe what takes place when you run out of them. It's called death. That's what dying means. There are no more metabolic enzymes to carry

314   Living Without Pain

out the functions of life, so life ends. That may be when you're 120, but they **will** run out. It would be as though when you were born, you were given a bank account that contained a certain amount of money for your entire lifetime from which you could remove, but not add, money. You can either be prudent with that money and make it last a long time, or you can squander it and let it run out sooner than you wish.

So it is with metabolic enzymes. It's an extremely simple equation. The more metabolic enzymes you require and use up, the unhealthier you will be and the shorter your life will be. The fewer metabolic enzymes you require and use up, the healthier you will be and the longer you will live. And of that, there is simply no doubt. Anything, and I mean **anything** you can do to use up fewer of your metabolic enzymes is obviously one of the most intelligent and life-enhancing practices you can cultivate as regards your health and longevity.

The second type of enzymes are digestive enzymes. As you learned in Step Three To Recovery, these enzymes are involved in the specific job of digestion. Food in the stomach is a Number 1 priority for the human body, and digestive enzymes are required to perform the process of digestion of food in the stomach. Pretty simple stuff.

Now, right here I would like to jump to food enzymes, which are the third type of enzyme, as a discussion will clarify the role of digestive enzymes. All food that has grown out of the ground, as part of God's grand scheme of things, has contained in it all the necessary enzymes to break it down in the body for digestion. Before going into the immense importance of food enzymes, I need to give you some corollary information that will help you more fully appreciate the importance and significance of not only food enzymes but also digestive and metabolic enzymes.

There are many elements that set humans apart from all other animal species on the planet. One of the more impressive differences is our more highly developed brain and our ability to think and reason. It is what allows us to accomplish so much of what is not even in the realm of possibility for all the other so-called lower animals. Ironically, it is also what gets us into trouble as regards our health and well-being, trouble that the lower animals don't have to contend with, trouble that is associated with diet, nutrition, and health. For example, do you realize that we humans are the only species on earth to cook our foods before we eat them? We are also, not coincidentally, the only species to suffer from the diseases of affluence discussed earlier, which are heart disease, cancer, diabetes, osteoporosis, and obesity. Food keeps us alive; that is a simple, self-evident fact. Stop eating and you die. But way back in history, we started cooking the life out of our foods before eating them and we have been paying the price with pain, ill health, and premature death ever since.

Animals in nature do not ever eat cooked food and they do not suffer from the diseases of affluence. There are, of course, exceptions to this, but those exceptions come into play only as other animal species come into close contact with humans. And the closer the contact, the more disease occurs. For example, animals in zoos or animals we take as pets, or animals that are in some way forced to interact with humans, suffer from the same diseases of affluence that afflict humans. Because we feed them our cooked food! Could anything on earth be more obvious?

I must share with you one phenomenally impressive study that is recognized the world over as one of the most convincing studies on this subject ever conducted. I lived in Los Angeles for thirty-five years, so I did the bulk of my research at the UCLA Medical Library, one of the best in the country. I spent hundreds of hours there poring over studies to substantiate much of my work. Obviously this was before computers took over the world. Finding this amazing study, which I referred to briefly in the Introduction to Part Two, was like finding a winning lottery ticket. The study has come to be known as Pottenger's Cats.

Dr. Francis Pottenger carried out a meticulous, thorough, ten-year experiment using 900 cats placed on controlled diets. Only two items of food were used and were given either in their raw or cooked state. The results were so overwhelmingly conclusive and convincing that there can be no doubt whatsoever of living, uncooked food's superiority over cooked food. The cats fed only the living, raw food produced healthy kittens year after year. There was no ill health, no disease, and no premature death. Death came to those cats only as the natural consequence of old age. However, the cats fed on the same food, cooked, developed every one of humanity's modern ailments—heart disease, cancer, kidney and thyroid disease, pneumonia, paralysis, loss of teeth, arthritis, difficulty in labor, diminished sexual interest, diarrhea, irritability so intense that the cats were dangerous to handle, liver impairment, and osteoporosis. The excrement from these cats was so toxic that weeds refused to grow in the soil fertilized with it, whereas weeds proliferated in the stools from the cats fed the living, uncooked food. Here is the clincher: The first generation of kittens born to the group of cats who were fed only cooked food were sick and abnormal. The second generation was often born diseased or dead. By the third generation the mothers were sterile. Dr. Pottenger conducted similar tests on white mice and the results coincided exactly with those of the tests run on cats.

So what do Pottenger's Cats and cooked food have to do with my discussion of enzymes? Just this: Far less heat than is required to cook food entirely obliterates all food enzymes. I want to be certain that you are clear on what I am saying. When you cook your food, the enzymes necessary to break down that food in your body are destroyed. Not **some** of them; **all** of them. And they're not merely degraded or made to be less effective. They are, every last one, completely and totally wiped out. This sets up quite a predicament for your body; one that has some very negative results. You see, food in the stomach, as I said, is a Number 1 priority for your body. Food can't simply sit around in your stomach; it has to be dealt with immediately. But if the food has been cooked, the enzymes that would have done that job are gone.

At this crucial moment, the wisdom and intelligence of the body snaps into action and calls upon the mechanism in the body that produces metabolic enzymes and forces it to produce the digestive enzymes necessary to digest the food. Now remember, this mechanism that produces metabolic enzymes is the very same one that determines the length and quality of your life. We know that this mechanism can only produce a certain number of enzymes, and then life ends. So every time you eat something that is cooked, you are literally inviting ill health and shortening your life.

The reason this is so is that when you suddenly force the metabolic enzyme mechanism to produce digestive enzymes, the work that the metabolic enzymes would have been doing to keep everything working efficiently and effectively, thereby keeping you well and healthy, is compromised and thwarted. The very mechanism in the body designed to keep you healthy and energetic is kept from doing its job. If your lymph system is overburdened, that means your body is working to decrease the amount of waste that has accumulated, which can ultimately cause you pain and make you sick. Every time you eat cooked food, you not only lessen the effectiveness of your body's labor force (metabolic enzymes) that is trying to cleanse and strengthen your body, but you also rob unnecessarily from the very mechanism that determines how long and how well you will live. And that has to be the last thing on earth you would ever want to intentionally do.

Right about now you might be thinking that I'm getting around to convincing you to become a total raw fooder, eating only uncooked food. Nope! That is not my intention. Hey, I like cooked food and I'm not about to give it up. So I'm sure as heaven not going to suggest that you do. Now, without question, the amount of uncooked food I eat does far outweigh the cooked food I consume, but no, I'm not going to suggest that we stop eating all cooked food. But here is what I am going to suggest, and it is the very purpose of these few pages.

Thanks to technological advances that did not exist when I wrote FIT FOR LIFE, there are now available

to one and all what are called live plant enzymes,
which can be taken just prior to eating anything
cooked, that do the job that the cooked-away enzymes
were supposed to do. They come in very small capsules, they are totally nontoxic, they have no side
effects other than increased health and longevity, and
they prevent the unnecessary squandering of your precious metabolic-enzyme capacity. These pharmaceutical-grade, live plant enzymes are grown and harvested
in a laboratory setting without compromising them
with heat or chemicals. In my opinion, the ability to
make these live plant enzymes available to us is one of
the most significant and beneficial advances of the
twentieth century. If there is a substance that could
rightly be called the fountain of youth, this is surely it.

From the day I found out these live plant enzymes
were available, until now, I have been taking them
whenever I eat anything cooked. No matter where I
am, no matter who I'm with, no matter what I'm
doing, I always carry them with me and take them
before eating any cooked food. At this point in my life,
I would just as soon pass on eating than to eat something cooked without my enzymes. I'm serious. I simply don't eat anything cooked if I don't have my
enzymes with me, and as much as I love to eat, you
can be sure that if you run into me somewhere, I'll
have capsules with me. If I don't, then you can be just
as sure that I'm not on my way to a restaurant, unless,

of course, I plan on eating salad or something else that has not been cooked.

I did some research into which enzymes were the absolute finest, purest, most high-quality live plant enzymes available anywhere in the world, and those are the only ones I take. Consider the words of Dr. Edward Howell, the man considered to be the father of enzyme nutrition:

"I like to think of life as an integration of enzyme reactions. Life ends when the worn out metabolic enzyme activity of the body machine drops to such a low point that it is unable to carry on vital enzyme reactions. This is the true trademark of old age. Old age and debilitated metabolic enzyme activity are synonymous. If we postpone the debilitation of metabolic enzyme activity, what we now call old age could become the glorious prime of life."[59]

Allow me to ask you a question. Would there by any possibility at all, **any**, of you going to the bank on a regular basis, taking out your hard-earned cash, and then using it as toilet paper? Any chance at all? Can you even think of anything that would be more absurd and ridiculous? No? Well, I can. I can think of one thing more absurd than using your cash as toilet paper and that would be using up the metabolic enzymes in your body that keep you healthy, alive, and free of pain, in order to digest cooked food that you could have taken live plant enzymes for. If a long life free of pain, ill health, and disease is one of the goals you have for yourself and your loved ones then start using live plant enzymes now! Many people who have started using these digestive enzymes upon my recommendation, have reported to me that the bloated feeling they customarily experience after a meal has completely disappeared since the regular use of these enzymes. Others have told me that other digestive disorders that usually require some kind of digestive aid to quell the discomfort (gas, pain, heartburn, acid indigestion and reflux) have also disappeared. Do this for yourself—you're worth it.

Ten years from now the need to take live plant enzymes with cooked food will be as well established as today's dictum that to acquire and maintain a high level of health we must exercise and eat right. Don't wait! Take advantage of this information now and get a jump on it. You will be glad for the rest of your long and healthy life.

Now that the true worth and value of enzymes have been well established as a real and viable alternative to drugs, there have been some very encouraging developments. For one thing, first class companies now exist, run by people of the highest integrity, who have a genuine desire and dedication to produce enzymes of the absolute highest quality. One such company is Enzymedica, whose full line of products is available at most health food stores across the United States. I am personally acquainted with the people who oversee this company and their expertise and dedication is unrivaled in the enzyme industry. They don't just meet minimum industry standards but have as a resolute company policy that their finished product will be unsurpassed.

Today there are highly effective enzyme products that fully support the living body's ongoing effort to heal itself rather than further toxifying the body while putting it at risk of injury and death as do drugs. There are enzymes to help with Candida, improve gastrointestinal discomfort, lower fat and cholesterol, support immune function, break down mucous, normalize pH balance, and lactose digestion. Plus, there are two in particular I want to let you know about that actually assist the body in reducing inflammation.

Repair is a high-potency blend of *proteolytic enzymes* (enzymes that break down protein) that is intended to support circulation, reduce inflammation, and speed healing. The enzyme Bromelain in particular is known for its ability to reduce the symptoms of inflammation. This is because it becomes active in a temperature slightly above normal body temperature. Body temperature rises at the point of inflammation and Bromelain seems to be drawn to the area bringing with it the other enzymes. Once there, these enzymes help reduce inflammation by breaking down the proteins that restrict blood flow and slow healing.

Natto-K, which contains the newly discovered enzyme *Nattokinase* along with six additional enzymes and a blend of minerals known to support Nattokinase, was first discovered by a doctor in Japan. It has been shown to support and assist the only enzyme found in the body to remove blood clots. It is because of its ability to break down the protein structure of a clot that so much excitement has been generated, since no other "non-synthetic" enzyme has the ability to do this efficiently. In the past, pharmaceutical drugs have been used intravenously for this purpose immediately after a heart attack or stroke to prevent further risk and damage.

One of the major concerns of inflammation is capillary blood flow. These small blood vessels are responsible for carrying oxygen and nutrients to the cells and removing waste. When these capillaries become damaged, it renders them incapable of carrying fluid to and from the damaged tissue. The result is pain, swelling, redness, heat, and loss of function. By repairing the capillaries, the bruises, swelling and pain disappear. Proteolytic enzymes have been shown to reduce the amount of fibrin (protein that forms in the blood after trauma or injury) in the damaged capillary, improve circulation and speed healing. Once in the bloodstream proteolytic enzymes digest the fibrin network and enhance blood flow. Plus, these same proteolytic enzymes have been known to stimulate cells that ingest foreign particles and debris in the blood and accelerate elimination by way of the lymphatic system. Both **Repair** and **Natto-K** clear the blood, enhance blood flow, and help reduce inflammation. **Repair** works more in the joints and muscles while **Natto-K** improves the health of the cardiovascular system overall as it works more on the cellular level and in deep tissue.

You can find out how to order, or receive more information on, the entire line of enzymes, including Live Plant Digestive Enzymes, **Repair**, and **Natto-K** by calling toll free: 877-335-1509 or by going to our website: www.fitforlifetime.com.

APPENDIX II:

MINERALS FOR LIFE

Your body is able to manufacture some vitamins, but it cannot make any of the minerals that are necessary for life. You must obtain an abundant supply of food-grade minerals from your diet, and if you don't, all manner of health problems can result, both minor and major. Since most people I've known know precious little about minerals, I'm going to lay out a few interesting and pertinent facts about them. First of all, we still do not know all the minerals that are present and utilized within the body. There are between twenty-five and thirty that have definite and known uses and about a dozen more whose uses are not fully understood. There are some found in appreciable quantities within the body, including calcium, magnesium, phosphorous and iron. Most minerals are called "trace minerals" because of the minute amount present in the body, such as zinc, cobalt, silver and boron.

There is definitely confusion as to what type of minerals can and cannot be used by the body. Most knowledgeable people recognize that the body must have certain minerals to accomplish its work and preserve health. However, only a few realize that these minerals must be in their organic state to do us any good.

Here are the facts: (1) Minerals are inorganic as they exist naturally in the soil and water; (2) Minerals are organic as they exist in plants and animals; (3) Only plants or animals can transform inorganic minerals into organic minerals; (4) Animals are poor converters of inorganic minerals because they are engineered to get their minerals from plants or by eating other animals; (5) Inorganic minerals are only poorly absorbed (about 5%) and can be injurious to animals.

Because inorganic and organic minerals have the same chemical composition, they were confused by early researchers. They mistakenly assumed that a chemical similarity in minerals also meant there was a nutritive similarity. Big mistake. It's true that, chemically, iron in the bloodstream and iron in nails are the same, and that calcium in rocks (dolomite) is identical to calcium in the bones. But it is a grave error to believe that the body can digest, assimilate and utilize powdered nails and crushed rocks.

The number-one mineral, by quantity, needed by the human body is calcium. Calcium is biochemically necessary to life, crucial to health, and instrumental in keeping you flexible and youthful.

Over time, the average person becomes more and more depleted of calcium. By age forty, over 50 percent of Americans are severely calcium-deficient. These drastic declines show that the majority of Americans are not obtaining enough utilizable calcium from their diets. What I mean by utilizable is that it is in a form that can be absorbed and assimilated by the body. For that to occur the calcium must be "ionized," or it is worthless.

When minerals enter your body they interact with certain stomach secretions that render them capable of being absorbed. This process is called ionization. Every mineral you ingest must undergo ionization in your stomach before it can be assimilated. The body must reduce any form of dietary or supplemental calcium into calcium ions. These ion-charged particles of calcium are the only form of calcium the body is able to metabolize, and thereby absorb and have available for use.

If you don't obtain enough ionized calcium in your diet, especially from fruits and vegetables, the body will leach calcium from the bones, the only place it can, so it can neutralize acid. This leads directly to the dreaded osteoporosis.

The organic calcium in fruits and vegetables is already ionized, but most people don't eat nearly the amount of fruits and vegetables they should, so they resort to dairy products and/or calcium supplements. What could possibly be more obvious than the fact that dairy products and supplements simply are not the answer? Although Americans are one of the biggest dairy-eating populations in the world, they also continue to have one of the highest incidences of osteoporosis. Although the calcium in cow's milk is ionized from the cow, once it's subjected to the blistering heat of pasteurization the calcium is deranged and very little of it can be absorbed. Pasteurization kills and destroys everything of worth.

As far as taking calcium supplements, they are typically poorly ionized. For example, calcium citrate, made from crushed rocks, is only about 15% ionized. Calcium gluconate, also made from crushed rocks, is worse, only about 5% ionized. We are not rock eaters.

Trying to obtain the calcium your body needs from dairy products and supplements can have some very detrimental repercussions. Unfortunately, over the years, the mindset has been that taking in extra calcium from dairy or supplements is a harmless precaution. It isn't! In fact, it's disease-producing. Trying to fulfill the body's requirements for calcium with non-ionized calcium will not work. If your car requires premium, high-octane fuel and you fill the tank with diesel fuel, what do you think will happen? True, they're both fuels, but only one can be used by your car. It's not a harmless mistake. The car won't run, and the diesel will damage the engine.

The extra calcium that is not used by the body isn't harmlessly eliminated. It is picked up by the blood and deposited in the soft tissue—the blood vessels, skin, eyes, joints and internal organs. Unused calcium combines with fat and cholesterol in the blood vessels to cause hardening of the arteries. The calcium that ends up in the skin causes wrinkling. In the joints, it crystallizes and forms painful arthritic deposits. In the eyes, it takes the form of cataracts, and in the kidneys it forms kidney stones. Hardly a harmless practice. Are these maladies that I just listed not prevalent in the United States? Are they not right on par with our over-consumption of non-utilizable calcium?

There is another extremely important consideration that has to be taken into account, which over the years has been routinely misunderstood and overlooked. A mineral deficiency rarely exists in a vacuum. The study of minerals by themselves necessarily leads to a fragmented view of nutrition. Minerals have an inter-dependence with many other various elements of food and with the complex actions of the body itself. Minerals are not isolated food factors but rather parts of the nutritional whole. No mineral is used in isolation within the body. All minerals interact with other minerals.

This is so elemental as to stun the intellect; so few people grasp this simple but obvious fact of life. The way it has been set up by the intelligence that has been noted and praised throughout this book is that miner-als are created in concert with other cofactors in food and are intended to be ingested in that way. Still, owing in large part to the error of confusing organic, ionized minerals with inorganic, non-ionized ones because they are chemically the same, the habit of ingesting isolated, fragmented calcium persists.

If you've ever made rice, you know that the amount of water and amount of rice has a certain correct ratio. It is, in fact, a ratio of 2:1, or two cups of water for each cup of rice. If that 2:1 ratio is not adhered to, the rice will not come out properly. Too much or too little of either the water or the rice and you will wind up with rice that is either mushy and sticky or burnt and dry.

Would it interest you to know that in order for cal-cium to be effectively absorbed and utilized in the body, it has to not only be ionized but also must be in the presence of magnesium? It also requires certain trace minerals, but magnesium is the primary cofactor that calcium needs to be useable by the body. And the ratio of calcium to magnesium is the same as water to rice, or 2:1.

I can assure you that neither dairy products nor the vast majority of commercial supplements have calcium that is ionized or in the proper ratio of 2:1 calcium to magnesium. Even if certain calcium supplements have the correct amount of magnesium added, it is unlikely to be ionized. So on and on it goes, with Americans loading up on more than 125 billion pounds of dairy products a year and hundreds of millions of dollars worth of calcium supplements, and still problems associated with a calcium deficiency, most notably osteoporosis, are rampant. Is it working? No, it is not working, and proof that it is not is sadly right before our eyes.

I'm not writing this section for the sole purpose of loading you up with a bunch of bad news. Nor do I wish to leave you feeling hopeless that you can't help support the calcium needs of your body with a high-quality, nontoxic supplement that fully meets all the specific requirements necessary to be effective. On the contrary, I want to tell you about an amazing discovery that will surely revolutionize the entire calcium-supplement industry.

In 1979, a British journalist went to Japan to interview one of the oldest documented living people in the world, Mr. Izumi. He was a sprightly 115-year-old man in amazingly good health who lived on an island off the coast of Japan. He was healthy, active and alert. Many of the other inhabitants on the island were also in great health and seldom died before age ninety-five.

Researchers found the water the islanders drank was uniquely different. It contained ionized minerals leached from living coral on which the island was built. These unique coral minerals made the water highly alkaline. Drinking this water helped the body keep a superior acid-alkaline balance. If you will recall, earlier in the book I pointed out that the human bloodstream is slightly alkaline and must stay in the alkaline range. However, the American diet is highly acidic, so there is a constant need for the body to neutralize this acid, and calcium is leached from the bones to do so.

Because the living coral ingests a large spectrum of natural, sun-radiated minerals from the ocean water, powder made from the coral contains a rich concentration of these naturally occurring minerals. Here's the truly exciting part of this discovery: These coral minerals are the only source in the world of minerals that are naturally in a highly ionized state (up to 92 percent!). Plus, the coral's large amounts of both ionized calcium and magnesium naturally occur in the exact right ratio of 2:1. And if that were not enough, it also contains the necessary trace minerals such as zinc, copper and manganese, also in ionized form, and is free of toxic metals such as lead, mercury, cadmium and arsenic.

This favored species of coral also contains a harmless form of aluminum; this form of aluminum occurs naturally in the same form found in literally all fruits and vegetables (not the dangerous form found in toxic dental restorative materials and associated with memory problems).

I started to notice that these "coral calciums" were being aggressively marketed in magazines, infomercials and through multilevel marketing. Like everything else that is marketed to the public, I know that there are inferior and superior products of all kinds. I wanted to know which one of the coral calciums was the absolute, unrivaled best of the best, so I did precisely what I did when I wanted to locate the finest and purest Live Plant Enzymes: I conferred with the most knowledgeable and well-respected authorities in the world of nutritional research, those people to whom the experts go for dependable, definitive answers.

Did you know that research shows that you have only a 2.5% chance of selecting a nutritional product in the marketplace that is both nontoxic and effective? In other words, you have a 97.5% chance of selecting a nutritional product that is either toxic or doesn't work. This rather shocking statistic was confirmed in a landmark study reported in the *Journal of the American Nutraceutical Association* (Winter 1999).

If you are taking, or want to take, coral calcium, you should take several critical factors into consideration, and ask about them from whomever you are obtaining the product.

First, you should know that not all corals are equal; not by a long shot. There are 2,500 different species of coral worldwide with varying mineral contents and levels of ionization. Some contain calcium and almost no magnesium at all. Surprisingly, only one form contains naturally occurring magnesium in the ideal 2:1 calcium to magnesium ratio. Make sure you check the ingredients, and here's what to look for: Let's say, for example, in the ingredients listed it shows "calcium from coral-400 mg." That means since there is 400 mg of calcium there has to be 200 mg of magnesium. If it lists "magnesium source, such as magnesium corbonate-200 mg," it's not the best coral. The magnesium carbonate had to be added to bring the magnesium level up to the correct balance. The carbonate will not be ionized, so this would be an inferior product.

Also, you want to check to see if there are any flowing agents added such as silicone dioxide, which is sand, or magnesium stearate, which is toxic hydrogenated oil and creates Trans-fats known to cause elevated choles-terol levels. Deaths from heart disease and cancer have been reported to be highest among consumers of this type of fat.

You should also find out if the powder is ground by nickel-free grinders to retain the value of the coral and avoid any toxic nickel residues.

Find out also if isolated trace minerals have been added that have poor bioavailability. In the correct species of coral these are naturally occurring and high-ly bioavailable.

Last, vitamin D3 is essential for proper calcium absorption and it occurs naturally in the correct species of coral. If you see "vitamin D3 as cholecalcif-erol," you know it is synthetic.

The marine coral I researched meets all of these criteria, making it the finest coral-calcium product on the market today.

Ordinarily I would not encourage anyone to take a calcium supplement because I know that living food can supply our calcium needs and most calcium sup-plements simply do not make the grade. Since coral was once living, it thereby can transform minerals into an organic, highly ionized state. The fact is that the product I researched uses exclusively the species of coral that has the correct 2:1 calcium-to-magnesium ratio, and it is harvested and formulated under the strictest, most pristine conditions that result in a most superior product. For this reason I will tell you that if you wish to take a calcium supplement that is the purest, safest, highest-quality product available, this is the one in which you can have complete and total confidence.

You can find out how to obtain the coral calcium I have described here by calling toll free: 877-335-1509 or by going to our website: www.fitforlifetime.com.

NOTES

1. Findley, Steven, "Pain is our Number 1 Health Complaint," *USA TODAY*, Oct. 23, 1985.

2–4. "Pain In America: Highlights from A Gallup Survey," *Arthritis Foundation* website, accessed August, 2004.

5–8. "Pain In America: A Research Report," Survey Conducted for Merck by the Gallop Organization, 2000.

9. National Institute of Health, *The NIH Guide: New Directions In Pain Research*, Washington DC: GPO, 1998.

10. Finklestein, Joel B., "2002 Health Care Spending Hit $1.6 Trillion," *AM News*, Jan. 26, 2004.

11. Diamond, Harvey & Marilyn, *FIT FOR LIFE*, Warner Books, New York, 1985.

12. "Comparing Fibromyalgia Syndrome and Chronic Fatigue Syndrome," ImmuneSupport.com. accessed, October, 2004.

13. Griffin, E. Edward, *World Without Cancer*, American Media Publishing, May, 1996.

14. *Food, Nutrition, and the Prevention of Cancer: A Global Perspective*, American Institute for Cancer Research, 1997.

15. "Cancer Strongly Linked To Lifestyle and Diet," Reuters, Dec. 9, 1998.

16. "Study Says Obesity Causes 90,000 Cancer Deaths Each Year," The Associated Press, Apr. 24, 2003.

17. Zimmerman, Michael and Kretchmer, Norman, "Isn't It Time to Teach Nutrition to Medical Students?," *American Journal of Clinical Nutrition*, #58-1993.

18. "Antibiotics May Cut Heart Attack Risk," N.Y. Times News Service, Feb. 3, 1999.

19. "Drug May Hold Clues For Cancer," Associated Press, Feb. 15, 1996.

20. Hilchey, Tim, "Cancer Drug May Help Reduce Heart Ills," New York Times, Sep. 1, 1993.

21. "Blood Test May Help Detect Cancers Early," Sarasota Herald Tribune, Aug. 23, 1992.

22. "Gene Therapy May Help Battle Heart Disease," Associated Press, Nov. 16, 1994.

23. "Cow-cell Implants May Help Ease Pain," Associated Press, Nov. 17, 1994.

24. Starlanyl, Devin, M.D., and Copeland, Mary Ellen, M.S., M.A., *Fibromyalgia and Chronic Myofascial Pain Syndrome*, New Harbinger Publications, Oakland, Ca., 1996.

25–26. National Center for Chronic Disease Prevention and Health Promotion, Centers for Disease Control and Prevention, U.S. Department of Health and Human Services, Apr. 22, 2004.

27. "Introduction to Arthritis," The Arthritis Society, Dec. 5, 2002.

28. Shelton, Herbert S., *NATURAL HYGIENE: Man's*

Pristine Way Of Life, San Antonio, Tx., Dr. Shelton's Health School, 1968.

29. Berkow, Robert, M.D., *The Merck Manual*, Fifteenth Edition, Merck & Company, Inc., Rahway, N.J., 1987.

30. *The Incredible Machine*, The National Geographic Society, Washington DC, 1996.

31. "Here's Another View: Tobacco May Be Harmless," *U.S. News & World Report*, Aug. 2, 1957.

32. Guyton, A.C., M.D., *Medical Physiology*, W.B. Saunders, New York, 1962.

33. Dr. Susan Love, "The Breast Care Test," PBS-TV, Oct. 18, 1993.

34. "Drug Industry On A $125 Billion Roll," *Health Freedom News*, Jan./Feb. 2001.

34A. Clarke, Kevin, "Prescriptions for Disaster," *U.S. Catholic*, Vol.#69, No.#11, Nov. 2004.

34B. Pear, Robert, "Few Enroll in Low-Cost Drug Demonstration," *The New York Times*, Sep. 11, 2004.

35. Mathews, Anna Wilde, "New Vioxx Study Projects Cases of Heart Attacks," *The Wall Street Journal*, Oct. 6, 2004.

35A. "Report: Merck Tried to Bury Vioxx Concerns," *Reuters*, Nov. 1, 2004.

35B. "UK Warns of Dangers Associated with Arthritis Drug," *Health Talk (Canada)*, Aug. 2, 2004.

35C. Henderson, Diedtra, "Centocor Warns of Remicade-Lymphoma Risk," Associated Press, Oct. 7, 2004.

35D. "Arthritis Improves with Remicade plus Methotrexate," Reuters, Nov. 30. 2004.

35E. "Study: 2 Million Get Sick from Drugs," *Washington Post*, Apr. 15, 1998.

36. Pottenger, Francis M., "The effect of Heat-Processed Foods and Metabolized Vitamin D Milk on the Dentofacial Structures of Experimental Animals," *American Journal of Orthodontics and Oral Surgery*, Aug. 8, 1946.

37. "The Dismal Truth About Teenage Health," *Reader's Digest*, March, 1986.

38. "Overweight Teens Risk Heart Disease, Diabetes Later," *The Washington Post*, Aug. 12, 2003.

39. "In Vitro Screening Study of 196 Natural Products for Toxicity and Efficacy," *Journal of the American Nutraceutical Association*, Vol.#2, No.#1, Winter, 1999.

40. "Fibromyalgia, Definition and Incidence," *Nutramed.com*, accessed Sep. 28, 2004.

41. Hitti, Miranda, "Daily Pain, Fatigue from Rheumatoid Arthritis," *WebMD Medical News*, Oct. 1, 2004.

42–45. Lewinnek, George E., M.D., "The Significance and a Comparative Analysis of the Epidemiology of Hip Fractures," *Clinical Orthopedics and Related Research*, Oct. 1980.

United Nations Food and Agricultural Organization, *FAO Production Yearbook*, 37, 1984.

United Nations Food and Agricultural Organization, *Food Balance Sheets: 1979-81 Average*, Rome, Italy, 1984.

Walker, Alexander R.P., D.Sc., "The Human Requirement of Calcium: Should Low Intakes Be Supplemented?," *American Journal of Clinical Nutrition*, May, 1972.

Walker, Alexander R.P., D.Sc., "Osteoporosis and Calcium Deficiency," *American Journal of Clinical Nutrition*, Mar. 1965.

46. Campbell, T. Colin, M.D., et al., *Cornell-Oxford-China Project on Nutrition, Health and Environment, Diet, Lifestyle and Mortality in China: A Study of the Characteristics of Sixty-Five Countries*, Oxford University Press, The China People's Medical Publishing House, 1990.

47. "A Gene-Environment Interaction Between Smoking and Shared Epitope Genes in HLA-DR Provides A High Risk of Seropositive Rheumatoid Arthritis," *Journal of Arthritis and Rheumatism*, Oct. 8, 2004.

48. Yee, Daniel, "No Matter How Exercise is Defined, We Don't Get Enough," *The Associated Press*, Aug. 15, 2003.

49. Rippe, James M., Dr. James M. Rippe's Complete Book of Fitness Walking, Prentice Hall, New York, 1989.

49A. Nenonen, M.T., et al. "Uncooked, Lactobacilli-rich, Vegan Food and Rheumatoid Arthritis." British Journal of Rheumatology, #37(3), 1998.

50. "Bottled Water Watch," New Age Magazine, Jul/Aug. 1999.

51. Cohen, Elizabeth, CNN Medical Correspondent, *CNN This Morning*, May 24, 2004.

52. Chopra, Deepak, *Unconditional Life*, Bantam Books, New York, 1991.

53. Talan, L., "Good Thoughts—Good Health," *Sarasota Herald Tribune*, Jun. 12, 1991.

54. Oberleder, M., "Avoid the Aging Trap," *Acropolis*, Washington DC, 1982.

55. Chopra, Deepak, *Quantum Healing*, Bantam Books, New York, 1989.

56. Beecher, H.K., "The Powerful Placebo," *Journal of the American Medical Association*, Vol.#159, No.17, Dec. 29, 1955

Wolf, S., "The Pharmacology of Placebos," *Pharmacology Review*, Vol.#11, No.4, Dec., 1959.

Pogge, R., "The toxic Placebo: Side and toxic Effects Reported During Administration of Placebo Medicine," *Medical Times*, No. 91, Aug. 1963.

57. Brown, S., "Side Reactions to Pyribenzamine Medication," *Proc. Soc. Exp. Bio. Med.*, Vol.#67, No.3, Mar. 1948.

58. O'Regan, Brendan, "Healing, Remission, and Miracle Cures," *Whole Earth Review*, Winter, 1989.

59. Howell, Edward, M.D., Enzyme Nutrition, Avery Publishing, New Jersey, 1985.

INDEX

C

caffeine, 137–38
calcium, 250, 253–54,
    329–38. *See also* coral
    minerals
cancer
    diet and, 36
    drugs and, 118
carbohydrate intake, 209–10
cardiovascular system, 277,
    278
cartilage, 55, 57
Celebrex, 117
Champion juicer, 176–77
chiropractic, 264
chronic fatigue syndrome,
    14–17, 22–24, 58–60
    causes, 77–78, 103–4,
    113–14, 237–38. *See also*
    toxins
    development and clinical
    course, 121–22
    symptoms, 113–14
circadian rhythms, 194–95
cleanliness. *See also* elimina-
    tion; natural hygiene
    importance of, 67–69,
    73–74, 81
colds, 101–2
colon problems, 269–71
connective tissue, 54–58, 113,
    262

cooking. *See* digestive
    enzymes, live plant; raw
    vs. cooked food
coral calcium, 253
coral minerals, 305, 334–38
COX-2 inhibitors, 117–18,
    120

D

dairy products, 220, 246–53.
    See also Pottenger's cats
    experiment; protein foods
    pasteurization, 155, 330
detoxification, 179. *See also*
    elimination; mono-dieting
    symptoms intensifying
    during, 183–85
diabetes, 209–10
diet, 34–38, 144–46, 148–49,
    188–90. *See also* mono-
    dieting; specific topics
dietitians, 191–93, 198–199,
    213
Digest 90 Vcaps, 305
digestion. *See also* food com-
    bining
    energy required for,
    138–40, 164–66, 177,
    178, 198–200, 212,
    226–28, 237–38, 308–10
digestive enzymes, 314–15.
    See also enzymes
    live plant, 234–41, 321, 322
    selecting a brand of,

235, 239–41, 303,
305, 321–22
taking prior to eating
cooked food, 234–35,
239–42, 320–21
digestive problems, 142–44,
213–16, 237
causes, 227–28
drugs for, 142–44, 213–14
digestive system, 225,
228–29
limitations, 142
drugs, 43–45, 50–52, 84,
114–15, 118–20, 243–44.
deaths, 119
See also pharmaceutical
industry; specific disorders
prices, 116
used to suppress symp-
toms, 109, 114

E

eating experience, 141,
146–48
eczema, 271
elimination, 68, 69, 73–75,
78–84, 98–99, 269. *See
also* detoxification; lymphatic system
energy required for,
74–75, 78–79, 237–38
extraordinary means of,
100–102

elimination cycle, 195–204
energy. *See under* digestion;
elimination
Enzyme Nutrition (Howell),
234
enzyme-rich vs. enzyme-
depleted food, 150–53,
164, 171, 226, 230–31.
See also pasteurization;
raw vs. cooked food
Enzymedica products, 302–6,
322–23
enzymes, 311–25. *See also*
digestive enzymes
destroyed by cooking,
317–19. *See also* raw vs.
cooked food
metabolic, 313–14,
318–21
exercise, 256–60

F

fasting, 310
FEELING FIT FOUR kit,
304–6
FEELING FIT GREENS,
274. *See also* green superfood
fibromyalgia, 14–17, 22–24,
60, 113
causes of, 48–49, 73,
77–78, 103–4, 237–38.
See also toxins

medical doctors, 32, 37, 191, 295
  arrogance, 30, 32, 33, 37–38, 49–50, 110–11, 213, 223–24. *See also* "stomach virus"
medical knowledge, certainty regarding, 30, 37–38, 42–45, 49–50, 110–11, 213, 223–24, 242
medicine, conventional vs. natural hygiene, 71–72
mental health, 294–300
Methotrexate, 118
migraines, 262–63
milk. See dairy products
mind-body connection, 294–300. *See also* mental health
minerals, 327–38. *See also* calcium
  organic vs. inorganic, 328–30
mono-dieting, 167–69, 172–87, 222. *See also* food combining
  cautionary advice regarding, 182–85

N

National Pain Care Policy Act of 2003, 10–11

Natto-K, 324, 325
nattokinase, 324, 325
natural hygiene, 19–23, 34, 71–72, 214. See also cleanliness
natural hygienists, 33–34
nutrition, 34–38
nutritional supplements, 231–34. See also specific supplements and nutrients
  types and brands of, 239, 328–29, 335–37
nuts, 177–78

O

obesity, 191, 271. *See also* weight loss
osteoarthritis, 55–58
  nature of, 56
osteoporosis, 251–52, 330

P

pain
  causes of, 30, 103–4, 260–61. *See also* specific diseases
  costs due to, 10
  keys to overcoming, 139, 161
  prevalence of, 9–10